Cancervive

Susan Nessim and Judith Ellis

Cancervive

The
Challenge
of Life
After
Cancer

HOUGHTON MIFFLIN COMPANY

BOSTON 1991

For information about permission to reproduce selections from
this book, write to Permissions, Houghton Mifflin Company,
2 Park Street, Boston, Massachusetts 02108.

Library of Congress Cataloging-in-Publication Data

Nessim, Susan.
Cancervive : the challenge of life after cancer / Susan Nessim
and Judith Ellis.
p.   cm.
Includes bibliographical references.
ISBN 0-395-56190-6
1.Cancer — Patients — Rehabilitation.   2.Cancer — Psychological
aspects.   3.Self-help groups.   I.Ellis, Judith.   II.Title.
RC262.N476   1991   91-7710
616.99'403 — dc20   CIP

Printed in the United States of America

DOH 10 9 8 7 6 5 4 3 2 1

Cancervive® is a registered trademark
of Susan Nessim.

*For Lisa Jamison
and Lenore Ellis*

In the depth of winter I finally learned that within me there lay an invincible summer.

— Albert Camus

CONTENTS

5 Strong Bonds and Fragile Emotions:
Relationships with Family, Friends, and Significant Others 80

Recovery from Cancer: A Family Affair 81 • Cancer's Effect on Intimate Relationships 93 • Cancer's Effect on Friendships 100 • Cancer and Dating 104 • People Who Need People 109

6 The Insurance Obstacle *112*

The Bottom Line 113 • Job Lock 116 • Forced Out of the Work Place 118 • Caught in the Squeeze 119 • You Say Prosthetic, They Say Cosmetic 122 • Ways Around the Insurance Obstacle 127 • The Need for National Health Insurance 144 • Resources for Insurance Information 147

7 When the Résumé Includes Cancer *150*

Cancer's Stigma in the Work Place 151 • The Myths Behind Cancer-based Discrimination 154 • You, Your Employer, and the Law 156 • How to Deal with Work Place Discrimination 161 • Vocational Rehabilitation 172 • Turning the Tide 177 • Where to Go for Advice or Assistance 179

8 The Double-Edged Sword:
Long-Term Effects of Treatment 182

Pyrrhic Victories 183 • The Long-Term Effects of Chemotherapy 187 • The Long-Term Effects of Radiation 190 • Lymphedema 193 • Chronic Fatigue 198 • The Risk of Secondary Tumors 201 • When Anger Becomes a Long-Term Effect 204 • Living with Compromise 210 • The Importance of Follow-up 213 • Late Effects Clinics 215

THIS KIND OF book could not have been written a few decades ago; and yet it is a book that is long overdue. Until relatively recently, not many cancer patients survived their disease. But today more than half of them do, thanks to dramatic progress in the detection and treatment of cancer.

That's the good news. The bad news is that cancer survivors are unprepared for the ways in which their disease may continue to affect their lives long after remission. Up to now there wasn't a book that dealt exclusively with their unique needs. *Cancervive: The Challenge of Life After Cancer* fills the void by providing a compassionate, practical resource for and about life after cancer.

Until two years ago, I had never recognized the compelling need for such a book. The subject of cancer, not to mention the issues facing those who survived it, was completely foreign to me. That all changed in March of 1989, when I was diagnosed with kidney cancer. I received the news shortly after I'd completed a picture titled, ironically enough, *Dark Holiday*. Further tests revealed that my cancer had already metastasized to my lungs.

I was terrified, as was my family. The news threw us all into a panic — a controlled sort of panic, I might add, since we knew unrestrained fear was unproductive. The following week I checked into the National Institutes of Health in Be-

thesda, Maryland. Under the excellent care of Dr. Steven
Rosenberg I was prescribed an experimental protocol involving Interleuken II and alpha-interferon, followed by surgery to remove one of my kidneys. It was a fairly brutal but
extremely effective treatment. Within six months I was in
remission.

However, I soon found that being a cancer survivor was a
struggle of a different sort. There is always "it" hanging over
your head, and for me that's the hardest part. I also know
that while cancer treatment has evolved, social attitudes have
not. Cancer still carries a considerable stigma, which lies at
the root of many of the problems patients and survivors
encounter. But I wasn't about to let antiquated attitudes
hamper my recovery.

I have always been an intensely private person, yet I had no
desire to conceal the news of my illness. By sharing my story I
wanted to show that it's possible to conquer cancer and go on
to lead a full life. I felt that because I am in such a visible profession I might be able to allay some of the fear surrounding
this disease by providing others with a positive example.

In turn, I was overwhelmed by the outpouring of support
and compassion I received from complete strangers. The love,
advice, kindness, and generosity that flowed my way simply
astounded me; it renewed my belief in the intrinsic goodness
of people. In that sense, my illness was an extraordinary,
transforming experience.

During my recovery, I also found out how therapeutic it is
to talk with other survivors. As wonderful as they are, most
doctors don't know what it's like to be treated for cancer.
They may know intellectually the fear that cancer brings, but
they can't know it in their hearts. And it's on that level that
cancer survivors connect.

Soon after I'd finished treatment my publicist was contacted by Susan Nessim, the founder of Cancervive. The or-

ganization had chosen me as the recipient of its Victory Award for 1990, to be presented at the annual Cancervive fund-raiser. In my profession, trophies are forever being handed out in recognition of some outstanding performance or achievement. So when I was presented with the Victory Award, it seemed strange at first to receive recognition just for being alive — even though I was thrilled to have qualified. The award acknowledges the most challenging role of my career — that of cancer survivor. Of all the performances in my life, this is the one that counts the most.

Susan and I met for lunch and discussed the issues her organization addresses. I was shocked and distressed to learn about the social barriers and physical and emotional burdens many survivors have to deal with once they are ready to re-enter society. I'm fortunate enough to work in a profession that is tolerant of illness, and I haven't personally come up against overtly prejudicial attitudes. As I listened to Susan, I had trouble understanding how such discrimination could exist — and yet I know it does. I now realize that education and advocacy are just two of the ways survivors can fight back. These are the themes that this book champions. We need to show the world that it is possible to have a history of cancer and still be a happy, healthy, vital person.

Although *Cancervive: The Challenge of Life After Cancer* was written specifically for survivors, its usefulness extends beyond that audience. Health care providers and the family and friends of recovered patients will also find this book insightful and informative. Through the voices of actual survivors, *Cancervive* vividly portrays the very real problems they too frequently encounter. The book doesn't gloss over or euphemize those issues; it tackles them head on. And it does so in a wonderfully inspiring, engaging way, providing useful, authoritative information that will, I am certain, help all survivors gain back a sense of balance and control in their lives.

The audience for a book like *Cancervive* didn't exist a generation ago. If my most fervent hope comes true, by the next generation the need for this book will be obsolete. Until then, the burgeoning community of cancer survivors needs a chart with which to navigate their way back into society. *Cancervive: The Challenge of Life After Cancer* is that guide.

— Lee Remick
Cape Cod, 1991

ACKNOWLEDGMENTS

WE ARE GRATEFUL to the following individuals for their advice and support: Joanne Frankfurt of the Employment Law Center / Legal Aid Society of San Francisco; Patricia Ganz, M.D., director of the Cancer Rehabilitation Project at the University of California–Los Angeles; Daniel Green, M.D., department of pediatrics, Roswell Park Memorial Institute; Sandra Horning, M.D., assistant professor of oncology, Stanford University Medical Center; Julie Katz, M.D., director of the long-term effects clinic at Children's Medical Center of Dallas; Frank L. Meyskens, Jr., M.D., director of the Clinical Cancer Center at the University of California–Irvine; Richard Miller, M.D., of I.D.E.C. Pharmaceutical Corporation; Maureen Montone of the public relations department at Memorial Sloan-Kettering Medical Center in New York; consumer advocate Ralph Nader; Joe Neglia, M.D., assistant professor of pediatric oncology, University of Minnesota; Christine Perkins, M.F.C.C.; Edwin M. Perkins, Ph.D., of the biology department at the University of Southern California; Theodore L. Phillips, M.D., chairman of the department of oncology/radiology, University of California–San Francisco Medical Center; and consumer writer Wesley J. Smith.

Appreciation is also extended to Robert Lee of Triad Agency and Russell Galen of the Scott Meredith Agency for getting the ball rolling, as well as to Lee Remick for lending her support to this project.

A special debt is owed to our editor, Frances Tenenbaum of Houghton Mifflin, whose suggestions for improving the manuscript were insightful and invaluable.

We also want to extend our warmest thanks to the following family members: Joan Lisa Ellis, R.N., Andrew Klotz, José A. Nessim, M.D., and Herbert S. and Rose Weintraub. Also, this book would not have been possible without the unfailing love, patience, and support of our husbands, Steve Nessim and Claude Teweles.

Finally, we wish to express our deep gratitude to the many survivors who took the time and had the courage to share their stories with us. Their contributions gave this book life.

INTRODUCTION

WHEN I LEFT Stanford University Medical Center fifteen years ago after treatment for cancer, I wasted no time in charging back into life. My one desire was to put the experience behind me.

But it wasn't long before I discovered that although I was cancer-free, I certainly wasn't free of cancer. A series of personal incidents revealed that there was more to overcoming this disease than surviving the hardships of treatment. Instead, the end of treatment marked the beginning of a new and unexpected challenge: adapting to life after cancer.

Six years ago I started Cancervive, a Los Angeles–based nonprofit organization for recovered cancer patients, because I realized I wasn't alone in the problems I faced. Since then I've heard from thousands of survivors who also find that the struggle against the disease is only half the battle. Although their doctors advise them to get back to work and on with their lives, that isn't always as easy as it sounds.

On leaving the hospital or outpatient clinic, recovering cancer patients are faced with a bumpy transitional period as they learn to adjust to life without the intensive medical support they received throughout treatment. During this particularly vulnerable time, survivors encounter unanticipated difficulties such as anxiety over ending treatment, delayed stress reactions, the fear of recurrence, and a variety of other problems of adjustment which are an inescapable part of living with a chronic, life-threatening disease. In addition, some must learn to adapt to chronic pain or the loss of a body part, while others are at risk for long-term complications of treatment.

As they reenter the mainstream, recovered patients must frequently contend with such formidable cancer-related obstacles as employment and insurance discrimination, altered family relationships, loss of friends, and for some, loss of fertility. In short, cancer creates lifelong physical, emotional, and psychosocial changes. And because there is virtually no comprehensive support system in place for them, survivors are all too often forced to grapple with these changes on their own.

That, simply put, is my reason for writing this book. Previous books about cancer, centering on the immediate needs of patients fighting the disease, have emphasized modes of treatment, techniques for coping, and the issues of death and dying. But although these issues are urgent and undeniably important, they aren't always relevant to those who have moved beyond the patient stage. The needs of survivors are different but no less significant. *Cancervive: The Challenge of Life After Cancer* is the first book to focus solely on the special concerns of those with a *history* of cancer.

The book begins with my story as a survivor, highlighting the events that galvanized me to form an organization for other recovered cancer patients. The chapters that follow draw on the personal accounts of Cancervive members, revealing the troubles and triumphs of people who are finding their way through life after cancer. The names of the survivors interviewed for this book have been changed, and several of their stories are composites, drawn from the transcripts of individuals who shared similar problems. The guarantee of anonymity freed many of them to reveal the profound emotional turmoil that is so much a part of the legacy of cancer.

Interwoven with their experiences are the advice and observations of noted authorities, including doctors, oncology nurses, psychologists, and social workers — all experts in the field of cancer survivorship. The final chapter, which includes a brief sketch of how Cancervive was formed, stresses the importance of support groups to survivors.

The experiences recounted in this book do not always reflect the triumphant, happily-ever-after image of cancer survivors so often presented in the mass media. Life after cancer is rarely as neat and tidy as that. Rather, our stories show how, by working through the aftermath of cancer, survivors can derive new meaning and purpose from the experience and thereby close the circle on their recovery. Life after cancer may be inalterably changed, but in many ways it can also be more vital and rewarding. The stories of many of the survivors told in this book are testament to that reality.

Cancer survivorship is a growing phenomenon in this country. Approximately one million Americans are diagnosed each year with cancer. Of that number, half can expect to live disease-free five years or more.* The National Cancer Institute estimates the current number of survivors at six million, and that figure increases each year. As a result, the medical community, the media, and even Congress have begun to take notice of the complex array of issues confronting survivors. But despite greater public awareness and improved information, recovered patients still find that they must pick their way through the psychosocial land mines that dot the field of survivorship.

Cancervive: The Challenge of Life After Cancer is intended as a resource and a survival guide for the recovered patient, illuminating the obstacles survivors face and offering the insights, tips, and strategies they have found useful in overcom-

---

*The survival time that is traditionally designated to mean a "cure."

ing them. My hope is that this book will help survivors realize that they are not alone, and that the pain of loss, so inextricably bound to the cancer experience, holds the potential for immeasurable gains and growth.

1

Facing the Challenge: My Story as a Survivor

AS THE PLANE made its final approach into Pittsburgh, I peered out the window at the mosaic of shimmering lights below. From my aerial viewpoint I tried to form a first impression of the city I would soon be calling home. The pilot banked hard, and the soft diffusion of city lights suddenly gave way to the night sky. I sat back in my seat, closed my eyes, and focused my thoughts on the excitement that lay ahead.

With this trip, I felt certain I was finally free of the past and the threat it had once held for me. Four years earlier, at the age of seventeen, I had been diagnosed with rhabdomyosarcoma, a rare form of cancer that attacked the soft tissue in my right thigh. With that diagnosis I embarked on a yearlong medical odyssey, and learned firsthand what it meant to live with the imminent threat of dying. As grim as the experience was, I emerged from it with new eyes. The world was somehow more vivid to me, richer and more sharply edged. I was exhilarated with the simple joy of being alive.

But I was also a little scared. That night I was flying to Pennsylvania to meet my fiancé's parents. As significant as that ritual is for most people, to me it held an even deeper meaning. A commitment to marriage meant a commitment to the future, a personal acknowledgment that I was going to live and thrive. I'd finally put cancer behind me.

Michael, my fiancé, was at the airport waiting to greet me. We had met more than a year before at the University of Colorado–Boulder, shortly after I'd returned to college following cancer treatment. I was then a sophomore intent on getting a degree in business. Michael, a senior, was studying to be an architect. We were introduced through mutual friends, and in two months' time we were dating exclusively.

Michael and I were typical college kids, full of energy and enthusiasm for the future. He had no trouble accepting my medical history, nor did any of my friends. Although I'd had cancer, I didn't see how it could present any obstacles to the plans I envisioned. If anything, beating the disease had made me more resilient and confident in my abilities.

The fall semester arrived, and with it came the realization that Michael would soon be graduating. He planned to move back to Pittsburgh and join his father's architectural firm, where he would be groomed to eventually take over. But Michael and I were very much in love; there was no way we could be apart. We talked about a future together, and then one day, ring in hand, he proposed.

As the chill of winter settled on Boulder, I began to make plans for the wedding and our life together. Michael and I decided that after the wedding we would move back East and I would finish school in Pennsylvania. But I was apprehensive. I'd never even been to Pittsburgh.

"That's easy enough to arrange," Michael said. "Why don't you come home with me for Thanksgiving? You can meet my parents and get to know the city."

And so I found myself in Pittsburgh on a cold and moonless November night. As Michael drove away from the airport, I confided how anxious I was. "Just relax and be yourself," he said with a smile. "The rest will work itself out."

Although it was late when we arrived, his parents were waiting up for us. We sat in the kitchen and chatted. Michael and I talked excitedly about our plans for the weekend and the neighborhoods of Pittsburgh we hoped to scout for houses. His parents said very little, and I thought it odd. I'd always known Michael to be open and affable, yet his parents appeared cold and aloof. But I was tired and more than a little nervous, and so I dismissed those first impressions. I was sure a good night's sleep would give me a fresh take on my prospective in-laws.

The following morning, Michael's mother agreed to join us for a tour of the city. When we stopped at a restaurant for lunch, she and I sat alone for a few minutes while Michael parked the car. "Tell me," she said suddenly, "what's it like living with a time bomb inside you?"

The question stunned me. Was she joking? A look into her expressionless face told me that this was no attempt at humor. I didn't know what to do, how to answer her. I turned away, ignoring the remark, and frantically glanced around the restaurant for a sign of my fiancé.

But Michael's arrival did little to disperse the tension between his mother and me. As soon as we returned to the house I told him what had happened. His reaction surprised me. Instead of getting angry at his mother or empathizing with me, Michael responded with a dismissive shrug. "Oh, Susan," he said in his breezy manner, "you're being too sensitive. I'm sure she didn't mean anything by it."

Perhaps he was right. Although I was still upset, I was determined to let the incident pass.

That evening Michael's father took us all out for dinner.

Michael and his mother were engrossed in conversation when I turned to my future father-in-law and asked his opinion of our wedding plans. That question, I realized too late, was a mistake.

"You know, Susan, I'm sure you can understand my concern as Michael's father." He looked away sharply. "It's just that I don't want my son to be a widower."

In the abrupt and awkward silence that followed, I wondered what to say. But what could I say? I was afraid that if I tried to defend myself I'd fall apart. Instead I said nothing.

Once Michael and I were alone, I recounted my conversation with his father. Again he felt that I was overplaying the incident. I assured him that this was no exaggeration. But Michael could not, or would not, confront his parents. He continued to defend them, obliquely suggesting I be more grown up about it. I told him I wasn't comfortable staying in their house and would prefer to spend the rest of the weekend in a nearby hotel. I went upstairs to pack, hoping he would join me.

Instead, Michael remained downstairs with his parents. I finished packing my bags, slipped off my engagement ring, and placed it on the bedside table. Shattered and demoralized, I flew home the next day to Palo Alto, California, and my family.

At the time, Michael and his parents' behavior seemed incomprehensible and unforgivable. It wasn't until years later, when a mutual friend mentioned that Michael's uncle had died of cancer shortly before our engagement, that I began to understand the emotional subtext of that weekend in Pittsburgh. My fiancé had never mentioned his uncle's long illness, which had apparently taken a tremendous toll on the family. I now realized that Michael's parents wanted to protect their son from further pain, and in their eyes my medical history jeopardized his happiness. That in turn explained

Michael's actions — or more precisely, his inaction. He was undoubtedly afraid that our marriage would anger his parents and was paralyzed by the choice he had to make.

In the months that followed, I did my best to forget about Michael. I moved to San Francisco, where I took a job as a sales representative for a large cosmetics firm. It wasn't long before I struck up a friendship with Ellen, a young woman who also worked in the marketing department. As time went on, Ellen and I became fast friends; we were practically inseparable.

Our regional manager informed us that once we had completed our training we would be promoted and given our own territories to handle. I was looking forward to my promotion since I loved to travel. When a territory opened up in the Southwest, Ellen and I learned that the firm planned to cover it with someone from our office. The company was conducting interviews at its New York headquarters, so we both cleared our schedules for the trip.

"I've already booked a flight," Ellen announced when she dropped by my desk one morning. "I'm leaving the day after tomorrow. What about you?"

I couldn't leave until the following week. I wished her luck and told her not to be nervous.

I called Ellen the night she returned home, hoping to pick her brain about the interview. She sounded surprised to hear from me.

"So how did it go?" I asked.

She hesitated. "Well, I think I got the job."

"You mean they've already decided?"

"Yes. I guess they have."

I congratulated Ellen, but my enthusiasm was undeniably muted. Why hadn't I been given a chance to interview? The vice president of marketing had said he wanted to talk to both of us. What caused him to change his mind? I started asking questions and checking around. One day while having lunch with Kay, a company manager, I found the answer.

"I probably shouldn't even be telling you this," Kay began, "but it was such a lousy thing for them to do. I really thought you should know." She paused and leaned forward. "Ellen got the job because she told them you had cancer."

"You must be joking. . . ." My mouth was dry, and I suddenly found it difficult to speak. I was as confused by Kay's revelation as I was shocked by Ellen's betrayal. My bout with cancer had been years before. The success of my treatment appeared total, my long-term prognosis a relative certainty. My doctors had even used the word "cured." I simply didn't understand. How could cancer still be a factor in my eligibility for promotion? Kay must have seen the bewilderment in my face. She provided an explanation.

"Ellen said that because you'd had cancer and it had affected your leg, you wouldn't be physically able to handle all the traveling the job required."

Like a blow on a bruise, her words revived the pain and anger that I'd felt in Pittsburgh. How many years would have to pass before others saw me as a normal person? Of course I knew that cancer was a chronic illness; but then, so was heart disease. And yet, I told Kay, heart attacks weren't preventing many of the men we knew from getting ahead. Why should cancer be any different?

"The Big C scares most people," Kay observed. "They still think it's a death sentence, and they don't know how to deal with someone who's had it. If I were you, I'd keep my medical history under my hat. Save yourself the grief."

But Kay wasn't me, and she had never brushed up against her own mortality. I'd fought hard to beat cancer, and I was fiercely proud of my victory. Yet I knew that Kay was right. There were others who viewed my experience as a taint rather than a triumph. During my recovery I had made up my mind that I wasn't going to let the disease limit my goals and ambitions. But now, with a growing sense of outrage, I realized that cancer was continuing to reroute my life and cloud my future. And I wanted it to stop.

I knew I had to leave the company. My self-esteem had been eroded, and I didn't have the fortitude to fight back. I'm not sure I would have known where to start.

I eventually found another job promoting a new line of cosmetics. But I was no fool. When people at work inquired about my treatment-induced limp, I told them it was the result of a skiing accident. I hated having to lie about something of which I was in no way ashamed, but I knew all too well that the truth could sabotage me. So I tucked that part of my life away, concealing it from others as if it were a sinister offense.

During this time I met, dated, and later married a man named Richard. He was several years my senior and provided a solid, steadying force in my life. I looked up to Richard; in some ways he was like a father figure, protective and attentive. If anything, he was overly solicitous of my health and welfare.

But by our second wedding anniversary, the marriage was unraveling. During the preceding year I had gone through what I can only describe as a full-blown identity crisis. Unfortunately, Richard became an innocent bystander in my struggle with myself. I was now twenty-five and had no clear idea of who I was. Cancer had created fissures in my life that I'd spent years trying to cover up. Without my being aware of it, the disease had deeply affected my self-image. I knew cancer was a part of my identity, yet I felt tremendous pressure to deny that aspect of my life. I was strong, healthy, and ambitious. But was I really a "well" person if others — including my husband — saw me as less than healthy? And what if the cancer came back? Was I wasting my time planning for a future that might not happen?

It had taken me seven years just to begin asking myself

these questions, and as I sought answers the view I had of myself and my disease began to change. That, in turn, threatened Richard and inexorably altered the dynamics of our relationship. Richard viewed me as a dependent person, and when I'd first met and married him that's what I was. As I grew out of that role, we grew apart. Two and a half years after our storybook wedding, Richard and I divorced.

To help reestablish myself, I moved down the coast to Los Angeles. I was no stranger to L.A.; I'd lived the first eighteen years of my life there. I enjoyed being back among old friends and familiar haunts.

By my twenty-seventh birthday, my life seemed to be back on track. I landed a position as special events director for a large department store. The job was exciting, and I funneled most of my time and energy into it. I enjoyed a busy social life and began dating Steve Nessim, a good friend I'd known since high school.

Yet despite my progress I felt strangely unsettled. I couldn't seem to shake a pervasive sense of frustration and anger, an accumulation of unresolved emotions that I knew had their genesis in my experience with cancer. My old approach to dealing with the disease — to dodge and deny — didn't seem to be working anymore. My medical history had at various times undermined my employability, my insurability, even my marriageability. These repercussions were increasingly impossible to ignore or overlook.

The permanent damage caused by treatment fueled my anger. Cancer had altered my body image, and I had yet to accept and integrate those changes fully. I was also upset by my doctors' attitudes. They had saved my life, and for that I was thankful beyond words. But my gratitude didn't diminish the frustration I felt over their lack of support for my needs as a recovered cancer patient. When I tried to get answers to questions about the lymphedema in my leg (a chronic swell-

ing resulting from treatment-induced lymph node damage),
doctors would do little more than offer vague answers and re-
assurances. But I wanted more, I *needed* more than that.

A sense of isolation compounded my anger. I hadn't found
anyone in Los Angeles I could talk to about my problems as a
survivor. I started seeing a psychotherapist, and that helped.
But as understanding as she was, my therapist couldn't comprehend the inner turmoil I was experiencing. Friends were
no different. They were concerned, but I sensed that they
were also baffled. "Hey, you survived," they would chide me.
"You shouldn't be complaining. You're one of the lucky ones."
I couldn't argue with their logic. But it didn't solve my dilemma, and it certainly didn't dissolve or diminish my anger.

A friend suggested I look for answers in a cancer support
group. That made perfect sense to me. If I was going to find
empathy anywhere, I would find it among people whose lives
had also been touched by cancer. I attended one group, and
another, then a third. However, these groups were composed
of patients — people who were still fighting for their lives. My
needs were different. I had won that fight; now I was up
against different obstacles. No one, it seemed, could fully
understand the ripple effect cancer was continuing to have
on my life.

No one, that is, except Lisa. She understood because she
too was a survivor, though her battles were much more har-
rowing than mine.

I first met Lisa Jamison when I was eighteen, shortly after
finishing cancer treatment at Stanford Medical Center. Once
I had recovered enough to return to college, I arranged to
drive back to Boulder with an acquaintance. On the way, my
traveling companion suggested we stop in Lake Tahoe. She
had a good friend living there whom she wanted me to meet,
someone who had also recently completed cancer treatment.

Lisa and I hit it off immediately. She was my age and like

me had received treatment at Stanford. Lisa had been diagnosed at age fifteen with malignant teratoma, an ovarian cancer, and underwent two years of aggressive therapy. Now she
was in remission.

We spent hours comparing notes, talking about the doctors
we both knew and swapping war stories about our cancer
treatments. We also shared a wicked sense of humor. No subject was too macabre for us to poke fun at. We'd joke about
how, thanks to the effects of radiation treatment, we could
now get a tan in two minutes. Her sarcasm full throttle, Lisa
described how she used to rattle friends by telling them to
turn off the lights so they could see her glow in the dark.

As I left Lake Tahoe, Lisa and I agreed to stay in touch.
And we did, running up exorbitant telephone bills in the process. Lisa and I shared all that was transferable of our cancer
experience. We had both seen relationships change, career
goals become distorted, health insurance evaporate — all
because of cancer. We worried about recurrence, our pros-
pects for parenthood, and the long-term consequences of
treatment.

For Lisa, those consequences were already formidable. Her
cancer had been particularly virulent, and in a last-ditch
effort to turn the tide she had received an extremely high
dose of radiation. In her case, however, it had been too much
of a good thing; the radiotherapy had caused severe adhesions in her abdomen. Adhesions also affected the arteries in
her legs, progressively diminishing her ability to walk. Although she had many operations to repair the damage, no
doctor could offer permanent relief.

"I think my radiologist has a crush on me," Lisa would joke
from her hospital bed. "Why else would he have rigged it so I
have to come back here all the time?" Lisa had a marvelous
gift for disguising adversity, but sometimes the painful or-
deals would overwhelm her. "If this is the cure, give me back

the disease," she once remarked, her voice etched with bitterness. But those moments were few and far between. Even during her darkest times, Lisa's irrepressible optimism would eventually burst through the gloom.

But I was alarmed. Why hadn't Lisa been warned that these complications might arise? What sort of long-term effects of treatment might *I* expect somewhere down the line? The need for answers consumed me. I scoured libraries for books, articles, reports, anything that would shed light on our concerns as survivors. Nothing came close to providing adequate information. Every book I read on cancer dealt with the immediate needs of patients fighting the disease, detailing modes of treatment, emotional coping, and the issues of death and dying. But what about people who were living *after* cancer? Scores of books existed on the lifestyle problems faced by cardiac patients, diabetics, and alcoholics. Why weren't there similar books providing practical, long-term support for cancer survivors? I told Lisa about my futile search for information. "It's as if we'd been dropped in the middle of a desert," she observed, "and left to fend for ourselves."

By 1985 Lisa's health had further deteriorated and she was back in the hospital, this time for a colostomy. I felt helpless watching her struggle through yet another operation, but I did what I could to cheer her up. "When you're back on your feet," I told her, "let's plan a vacation together. Somewhere sunny and warm, where we can kick back and relax."

Two months later, Lisa called me from San Francisco. "Palm Springs," she announced. "You suggested we take a trip together, and I'm ready to go. Next weekend, okay?"

It was the perfect prescription. The hot dry weather lifted Lisa's spirits and seemed to help her feel better physically. On our first day in Palm Springs we talked long into the night about our lives and hopes for the future. As always, our conversation inevitably circled back to the subject of surviving cancer. As we talked, we vented our frustration. Why wasn't anyone addressing these issues?

Lisa reminded me. "Susan, you have to remember that the medical community is geared strictly toward treating the disease, not what comes after the cure." Between sips of iced tea she added, "If we want answers, we may have to provide them ourselves — or at least start the discussion. I think it's time we stop complaining and start doing."

I knew she was right. If we couldn't find a support group for survivors, we would have to create one ourselves. On the spot, Lisa and I decided to join forces and do just that. We began brainstorming, imagining an organization that would provide its members with peer support groups, professional counseling, and educational programs. Membership, we decided, would be open to people aged sixteen and older who had finished treatment, were considered disease-free, and were now trying to ease back into normal life.

We continued our brainstorming session the next day. Lisa sat in the hot desert sun, all but hidden under a big floppy hat, a yellow legal pad propped on her knees. On her notepad she outlined our goals and jotted down objectives, giving shape and structure to our ideas. Many hours and legal pads later Lisa abruptly looked up at me and said, "Cancervive. Let's call it Cancervive."

By the end of that weekend we had laid the groundwork for our new organization. We drove back to Los Angeles, and Lisa flew on to San Francisco. We were feeling exhilarated and hopeful, both of us eager to get started on making our weekend dream a reality.

Then tragedy struck. On her return home, Lisa's complications flared up and she was forced to reenter the hospital. The massive dose of radiation she'd received was now causing the major arteries in her pelvis and legs to close off. First a foot had to be amputated, then her entire leg. Several months later, doctors removed the other leg. I flew up to San Francisco, devastated by what had happened to my friend. I was also terrified. How could I be sure that what was happening to Lisa wouldn't one day happen to me?

Lisa saw the fear in my eyes. "Don't worry, Susan, you're going to be okay. After all, I'm counting on you to get Cancervive going." Then she smiled. "Just promise me you'll hold on to that leg of yours, all right?"

Lisa's ferocious fighting spirit gave me the inspiration I needed. I returned to Los Angeles and immediately started organizing the paperwork and getting the word out about a newly chartered nonprofit organization called Cancervive. I contacted newspapers, magazines, television stations, and hospitals. I was sure that hundreds, perhaps thousands of survivors were encountering problems similar to those Lisa and I had faced. It was just a matter of reaching them.

A few weeks later I was asked to appear on a national television talk show. The simple act of telling my story had an amazingly cathartic effect, not just on me, it seemed, but on other survivors who saw it. After my appearance the station was swamped with calls from survivors who had telephoned to say, in essence, "That's me. That's my life. Just change the name."

Lisa and I were elated by the response. We knew then that our reasons for starting Cancervive were valid.

I decided to keep the first support group meeting small and informal so that those attending would feel comfortable about speaking their minds. The group that gathered in my living room on a warm July evening in 1985 included two oncology social workers; Nancy, an eight-year survivor of Hodgkin's disease; and Jon, a young man who had finished treatment for a brain tumor six months before and was now in remission. I had no agenda planned. Instead, I suggested that we talk about our experiences as survivors, raising any and all issues that concerned us.

At first it was hard for Jon and Nancy to talk about themselves. Jon explained why.

"I'm uncomfortable talking about the negative aspects of surviving," he said. "I certainly don't want to sound like some kind of ingrate."

"That's okay," I responded. "Then if you don't mind, I'll start." I talked about my life, my bout with cancer, and the problems I encountered once I'd left the hospital. It wasn't easy speaking to a group of strangers, confiding some of my deepest fears and relating the pain and anger I'd kept bottled up inside for ten years. And yet, even though I hardly knew these people, I felt they weren't really strangers. They seemed to understand what I was saying and how I was feeling in a way only a survivor could.

"I don't think I'm alone," I said in conclusion. "I think these issues affect all survivors in one way or another, regardless of age or prognosis. I'm worried that other people will go through what I went through, and that they may take too long, as I did, to come to terms with the legacy of their cancer."

The room was silent for a few moments. Then Nancy spoke. "My boyfriend and I have talked about maybe getting married in a year or two, and it's made me think a lot about whether or not I can have children. I recently asked my doctor about it. He said that treatment probably left me infertile. It took a while for that to sink in, but once it did, I cried for days. Now I'm wondering, how do I tell my boyfriend? I'm so worried that it will change everything."

Jon nodded and said, "Now that I'm in remission, I can't stop thinking about a recurrence. With my kind of cancer, there's a good chance of that happening. My doctor says I shouldn't worry about it, that I should just put it out of my mind and get on with my life. But he isn't offering me any guarantees of a cure either. At least when I was getting radiation, I felt I had some protection. Being off treatment scares the hell out of me. I keep waiting for the other shoe to drop. How am I supposed to deal with that?"

I knew there were no easy answers to Jon's question, or Nancy's, or mine. But as we talked, a bond began to form among the members of this tiny nucleus of a support group. The more open we were about what had happened to us, the more unburdened we felt. I could empathize with Nancy's dilemma because it was my concern as well. I knew Jon's fear because I had faced it too. Our lives touched and crossed at a juncture called cancer, and it was there that we recognized ourselves in each other.

This was the beginning of Cancervive, the organization Lisa and I hoped would represent the needs and concerns of all survivors. The problems that Jon, Nancy, Lisa, and I faced weren't unique; they were just a few of the challenges that form the backdrop to life after cancer.

2

Returning to the Well World

I celebrated my twenty-first birthday as a cancer patient at the University of Texas M. D. Anderson Cancer Center in Houston. My parents threw a party for me in the hospital, and we asked everyone on my floor to attend. But we were celebrating more than just my birthday. The day before, my oncologist had presented me with the best present of all: he told me I was in remission.

I couldn't wait to get home, gain back my strength, and get on with my life. But a funny thing happened on my way back to the well world. Several weeks after leaving the hospital, I couldn't seem to shake a growing sense of anxiety. The care and support I'd received during my hospital stay had provided me with a sense of security. But now, on my own, I felt disoriented, frightened. I wasn't sure how to fit back into the outside world anymore.

— Anita, three-year survivor of osteosarcoma

REMISSION: no other word is as liberating and exhilarating to the cancer patient. Remission often means an end to the grueling round of treatments and tests, of countless visits with the medical team. It signals a return to health and the welcome reappearance of hair and energy. And best of all, remission means gaining back a sense of normality and getting on with life.

Or does it? Although this transitional period is outwardly a happy, celebratory one, survivors frequently find their joy tempered by unanticipated problems and emotions. When Anita shared her story with a Cancervive support group, we could immediately identify with her experience. Like Anita, many survivors leave the hospital with ambivalence, frightened and overwhelmed by the idea of stepping back into everyday life. They soon discover, as I did, that safe passage back to the well world isn't as easy as simply walking out the oncologist's door.

The road to recovery can be pitted with potholes, and some survivors wonder why they were never warned. One reason is that the psychosocial education of the recovered cancer patient is a relatively new field. Until recently, health professionals assumed that the only post-treatment hardships cancer patients had to endure were physical in nature. But with the dramatic increase in survival rates, it has become apparent that the psychological consequences of the disease are at least as important as the physical ones.

Dr. Michael B. Van Scoy-Mosher, an oncologist at Cedars-Sinai Medical Center in Los Angeles, is one of the growing number of doctors who concur with this view. "A lot of physicians feel that once cancer treatment is complete, the patient's problems are over and life goes on," says Dr. Van Scoy-Mosher. "But some of the greatest problems I've seen actually *begin* then. From my standpoint, the survivorship phase is one of the most challenging and in many ways the most difficult periods in the cancer patient's life."

Dr. Van Scoy-Mosher adds that the immediate post-treatment phase is a particularly vulnerable time. For instance, it's not uncommon for recovering patients to feel enormous anxiety about going off treatment or parting ways with the hospital staff. Many survivors have difficulty regaining a sense of control and direction in their lives, whereas others struggle with delayed stress reactions to their cancer experience. Throughout this process of "normalization," the questions and concerns never stop percolating: "What happens now? How will I fit back in? How can I be sure the cancer is gone?" In this chapter you will meet several survivors who wrestled with these concerns as they made their break from the acute stage of cancer care.

Breaking Free of the Hospital World

When Robert, a college student now in his fourth year of remission, first came to our support group, he struck me as a very self-assured, confident young man. He described how during his year and a half of chemotherapy for Hodgkin's disease, his sights were set on the day he would be free from the world of needles, nurses, and nausea. But as Robert explained, when that time came he discovered that his relief was mingled with other, unexpected emotions.

I'd always considered myself pretty much of an "in-control" guy, and I'd never had a problem with separation anxiety before. But then again, I'd never had cancer. And I'd never been stuck in a hospital for so long.

It's ironic, because I'd always had a phobia of hospitals. I hated the idea of even visiting them. And then — *boom* — there I was, forced to be a patient. I couldn't wait to be rid of the place, all the bland food and round-the-clock tests.

As I approached the end of my treatment protocol, I was naturally relieved to be getting away from all that. But to my surprise, I was also upset by it. I wasn't so worried about the cancer anymore; in fact, my oncologist even wrote a guarantee on my insurance form stating that I wouldn't get a recurrence. What I did feel was strong separation anxiety as the medical team slowly started to withdraw their attention. I suddenly realized how emotionally dependent I'd become on the hospital staff, even the chemo. I tried talking to my oncologist about it but his attitude seemed to be, "Hey, I have lots of sick people to treat."

I know it sounds crazy, and I'm more than a little embarrassed even admitting it, but I felt as though I'd been discarded. I was angry about it and anxious, even panicky at times. I could handle those feelings during the day, but the nights could be tough.

Robert certainly isn't the only survivor who worries about parting ways with the oncology ward. Anita, the survivor you met at the beginning of this chapter, expressed a similar concern. To someone who has never experienced a serious disease, anxiety over leaving the hospital might seem odd or overblown. But even those who receive outpatient treatment can become psychologically dependent on the medical world. Many survivors readjust fairly easily to normal life, but others may be plagued for weeks or months by mood swings, low self-esteem, and an undercurrent of anxiety.

When you think about it, those feelings are quite normal, even predictable. After all, a cancer diagnosis transforms your life. It also transfers much of the responsibility for your well-being to a group of relative strangers. Over time these health care professionals become like a second family. With your cancer diagnosis as the call to arms, they united with you in the fight for your life. They saw you at your worst, and they were there to cheer your victories. So it should come as no surprise that you have, perhaps unconsciously, developed strong psychological bonds with them.

Julie Steckel is a licensed clinical social worker in Los Angeles who works with recovering cancer patients. She finds that it's common for survivors to feel ambivalent about leaving the hospital world.

There is quite a bit of retooling, psychologically speaking, that takes place once cancer patients leave the acute phase of treatment. For some, it's difficult to let go of the sick role and all of the dependency and attention that goes with it. Many survivors are worried about leaving the safe, secure hospital environment. They may feel they are being abandoned at an extremely precarious time by some of the very people who have been most concerned for their well-being. Often this concern is compounded by the fear of recurrence, which is usually most intense at this time.

Then again, many survivors have the problem of fitting back into their old lives. They are no longer caught up in the intense drama that a crisis like cancer represents, and so they need to shift their focus to normal everyday activities. But cancer has forever changed these people. They now find that they have to redefine their identity, and that can be intimidating. All these changes can result in anxiety, fear, depression, even anger.

LETTING GO OF TREATMENT

As unpleasant as cancer therapy can be, many survivors dread the day it ends. When the oncologist announces the end of treatment, a patient's first reaction may be one of anxiety. "How will I live without it?"

That's the question Cory keeps asking herself. The fifty-six-year-old neonatal nurse was diagnosed with breast cancer three years ago. A biopsy following her mastectomy revealed that the disease had affected eleven lymph nodes. It had invaded Cory's chest wall and metastasized to her liver and spine.

But a few weeks ago Cory's physicians told her that the long, intensive course of chemotherapy and radiation had worked; her cancer was in remission. She recently talked to me about her ambivalence over ending treatment.

I've been on chemotherapy for three years now. Other than barfing up my insides all the time, I think I handled it pretty well. Now my oncologist tells me that I can quit chemo soon. He thinks it's great news, and I do too, except that I'm also scared to death. Chemo has been my security blanket. After all, it's a rare instance when a patient experiences a recurrence while receiving chemotherapy.

This isn't the first time I've faced this fear. After my second year of treatment, I was told I could probably go off it soon. Then my doctors took another look at my tests and decided that, just to be sure, I should get another year of chemo. I heard that and all I could think was, Oh, good! I don't have to worry about dying for another year. Chemo has almost become a way of life for me. I feel like an addict. Next month is my last month of treatment. I don't know how I'm going to handle it, knowing that I won't have those chemicals blasting away at any stray cancer cells.

Robert experienced a similar problem when he ended his treatment for Hodgkin's disease.

I first started noticing what I call my "withdrawal symptoms" right after my last chemotherapy treatment. When it came time to quit, it was just like going cold turkey. I really believed the treatment was all that was keeping me alive. I guess that's what was so psychologically addicting about it. It took me a while to realize that *I* had been just as important in the fight against my cancer as those drugs.

Recovering patients frequently use expressions like "cold turkey" and "withdrawal symptoms" when describing the psychological rigors of going off treatment. Some patients actually request that their treatment be prolonged, even though there is no medical reason for doing so.

As anxiety-provoking as the termination of treatment can be, keep in mind that too much medicine is as bad as too little. "Patients need to realize that everything we are currently using to treat cancer comes with its own set of problems," asserts Dr. Richard J. Steckel, director of the Jonsson Comprehensive Cancer Center at the University of California–Los Angeles.

The aim of oncology today is to balance any harmful side effects with the goal of getting the patient into remission. It is common for patients to feel that their treatment is their only real defense against cancer — that without it, there is nothing fighting the disease. But surgery, radiation, and chemotherapy often serve only as a means of pushing the balance of that fight in favor of the body. When all is said and done, it is the patient's own body that ultimately wields control over cancer.

Then again, termination of treatment signals an end to the reassuring routine of hospital surveillance. During treatment, you may have felt as if your lifeline was hooked to the alien, antiseptic world, and so the hospital became a haven offering womblike security. But no one can stay in the womb forever. Sooner or later, you have to start living the life cancer forced you to put on hold.

So how do you go about disengaging yourself emotionally from the hospital world? Several Cancervive members have succeeded by simply throwing themselves back into everyday activities. You might try to do this by quickly reestablishing old patterns and routines in your work, school, or family life. Focus on activities you enjoy or find worthwhile so that you can feel as if you are reinvesting yourself in the well world. Another way to allay anxiety is to protect your new-found health through a change in lifestyle habits. Cory decided on that approach:

I realized I could freak out over my withdrawal from chemotherapy, or I could take an active part in building myself up and bolstering my immune system. During the last year or two I've become very interested in how diet, nutrition, and stress seem to influence the body's immune response to diseases. I read somewhere that more than seventy percent of cancers are due to lifestyle habits. So I've made a concerted effort to change a lot of my old habits. No more high-fat foods, no more couch potato routine. I'm even learning how to meditate. I guess you could say I've adopted a holistic approach to the way I'm going to live my life. My kids think it's fantastic. I'll admit it hasn't been easy — I still sneak an occasional ice cream cone — but it is giving me a new sense of being in charge of my life. It also gives me peace of mind to know that I'm doing the best I can. The rest I'm just going to have to leave to the man upstairs.

Anita found that her anxieties were best addressed in group therapy. She says that the feedback, support, and camaraderie of other survivors kept her from falling into a state of helplessness. It also provided her with a few tips on how to handle her fears.

The first step for me was to face up to my feelings. By talking to other survivors, I discovered that I wasn't the only person who felt scared and disoriented after being released from the hospital. I was so relieved to know that it was okay to have those feelings. One of the people in my group said that the way she took care of her "remission blues" was to do hospital volunteer work once a week. Those weekly visits to familiar surroundings somehow reassure her and allow her to feel as if she's in control of the situation. I think I might try doing that.

Robert's approach to post-treatment anxiety was through yet another route:

I decided to drop in on one of the social workers I'd come to know during my treatment. I talked to her about the trouble I was having psychologically weaning myself from chemotherapy and hospital care. She suggested that since my oncologist wasn't very receptive to my problem, I should try talking to one of the other doctors on my treatment team. Ultimately, I did connect with another oncologist — a colleague of the guy who treated me. Although this oncologist had not been involved in my treatment, he knew my case and all the details. But more important, he was very receptive to my concerns. He said my anxiety was normal and that in time it would diminish and disappear. We talked about the specifics of my follow-up schedule and the particular symptoms I should watch for. In the meantime, he suggested I call him whenever I needed to talk, or as he put it, "plug in." His advice helped a lot. Now the time between my three-month checkups doesn't seem like an eternity. And what's more, I'm back to getting a good night's sleep.

One of these methods may work for you, but they are certainly not the only means available. You may find, as I did, that the simple act of talking about your anxieties with someone else can be wonderfully therapeutic. A survivor support group like Cancervive offers a forum where these concerns can be addressed and where coping techniques are shared. If you're not comfortable in a group, ask a friend or relative to lend an ear. But if you are having a particularly tough time readjusting after treatment and your anxiety is especially acute or prolonged, don't hesitate to seek professional help.

Renegotiating the Patient-Doctor Relationship

It is natural for recovered cancer patients to feel emotionally tied to the hospital when it has provided them with the medicine and machinery for successfully treating their disease. But occasionally survivors find themselves struggling with a more personal kind of bond, the traditional patient-doctor relationship.

Physicians have long held a revered place in our society. Many of us were brought up to believe that doctors can do no wrong — that they are beyond reproach, even beyond questioning. We see them as the captains and kings of our health, and when we are sick we depend on them to marshal the forces of modern medicine on our behalf. Who are we to doubt them?

Although this view is still widespread, it is changing. Most people now realize how essential it is to approach medical care as informed and responsible consumers. After all, oncology is a business — big business. Without you and consumers like you, the machinery of this multi-billion-dollar industry would grind to a halt. You have the right to ask questions, expect answers, and make health care decisions accordingly.

It is important to think of the relationship between doctor and patient as a partnership in which both parties have equal say in the decision-making process. As in all relationships, trust and communication are the essential ingredients.

According to Dr. Van Scoy-Mosher, there are two extreme versions of the patient-doctor relationship:

At one end of the spectrum is the paternalistic approach, where the doctor is the authority figure. He makes all the decisions as to what the patient needs. The other extreme is that of patient sovereignty, where the doctor hands the patient a laundry list of possible choices and then lets the patient decide. Somewhere in between these two approaches is a relationship based on shared decision making.

Dr. Van Scoy-Mosher believes the oncologist's role is best described as that of a guide.

I'm not there to tell the patient what to do, but rather to guide the patient into making the right choices. This requires communication and a series of two-way commitments. Each of us, on either end of the stethoscope, should listen and develop empathy for what it's like on the other end.

But there are times when either the doctor isn't listening or the patient isn't communicating, and as a result, empathy is in short supply. Five years ago, a forty-nine-year-old Cancervive member named Dana underwent a modified double mastectomy. While she was recuperating, her surgeon told her that because there was no lymph node involvement she wouldn't require any follow-up treatment. But Dana's elation over the news was soon undercut by the anger she felt toward her doctor.

I went into the mastectomy operation counting on the surgeon to save my life. At that point, I trusted him implicitly. I thought he was like God, this omnipotent authority figure. And, of course, I was the typical passive patient.

After my surgery, just before I left the hospital, I asked my doctor what I needed to do from that point on. What should I watch out for? Was there anything I could do to control the swelling in my left arm? He answered rather brusquely, "No, not really. Just be sure to get a chest X ray every year." With that, he turned and left the room. I was completely stunned by his cavalier attitude. He had just cut off both my breasts, and he was treating me as if I'd had a mole removed. He could see that I was upset and scared. He knew I needed answers to questions. Instead he acted like a jerk. His interest was in the disease, not me, the patient. I felt as if I had been summarily booted out the front door. I wanted to respect and trust my doctor, but instead I felt betrayed.

Dana told me that it was her anger over this incident that prompted her to attend a Cancervive support group. Dana is no wallflower, and she used her first group meeting to vent her rage. She talked with other survivors and compared notes on their patient-doctor relationships.

I listened to a couple of other women describe their mastectomy experiences, and I suddenly felt like I had gone through mine with blinders on. They helped me see that although my mastectomy was performed by a competent surgeon, he also happened to be an insensitive and uncommunicative doctor. I slowly came to understand that he was, after all, only human. That diffused a lot of my anger and really opened my eyes to the kind of patient I had been. Now I'm no longer passive when it comes to my own well-being. I made the decision not to go back to this doctor for follow-ups. Since then, I've found a physician who has a terrific bedside manner. He really takes the time to listen and was tremendously helpful in guiding me to another surgeon for breast reconstruction. I'm finally beginning to appreciate how my cancer experience changed me; it made me more alert and self-reliant. And that in turn has affected my relationship with doctors.

As both Dana and Robert know, the termination of therapy can be an especially vulnerable time in the patient-doctor relationship. As the patient approaches the end of treatment, visits to the doctor's office take less and less time, until that last appointment. This meeting can be so short and cursory that many people end up feeling as if they have been somehow deserted, left alone to deal with the uncertainties of recovery. Says Julie Steckel:

Many times this is a reaction to the doctor's telling the patient in essence, "I've cured you. I've done my part in this joint victory; you won't be needing me as much anymore." This is often the doctor's way of letting go. However, because the patient is dependent on the doctor, he or she may experience the break as a personal abandonment — even a betrayal. The end of treatment is really the end of an era, so to speak, and one that needs to be acknowledged by both the patient and the doctor.

As it is, very few physicians learn how to handle the emotional dynamics that accompany the end of the patient-doctor relationship. This is not to imply that all physicians are insensitive to the emotional concerns of their patients. Many are very supportive. Nonetheless, the majority of physicians still believe that a patient's psychosocial problems are more appropriately the domain of social workers and other therapists. Also, because of the extraordinary demands of their profession, physicians frequently remain detached from the people they treat in order not to become emotionally overwhelmed by their distress. For many doctors, this coping mechanism is essential. But all too often, patients interpret such behavior as defensive, unresponsive, or uncaring.

I don't mean to suggest that whenever problems arise between patient and physician, the doctor is always to blame.

Like Dana, too many of us still adopt a passive rather than an active attitude when it comes to dealing with the medical community. As a patient, however, you need to realize that you have duties and responsibilities too. Don't forget that you are an integral part of the health care team; your input is essential. When lines of communication between patient and doctor aren't as open as they should be, both parties end up second-guessing each other, and misunderstandings can mushroom into crises. Of course, there will always be patients for whom ignorance is bliss. Some people simply cope better with few facts and plenty of faith. This is a perfectly acceptable approach, provided it works for and not against you.

Dr. Richard Steckel believes that at the end of treatment physicians should conduct a sort of "debriefing" session with their patients.

I think it's crucial for the patient, once finished with treatment, to sit down with the doctor and discuss the entire experience. In many ways it's just as important to leave the acute phase of treatment with the same kind of interview and review that the patient and doctor had at the time of the initial diagnosis or before treatment. It is particularly important for the patient to get as much information as he or she needs to ensure a successful recovery. Also, having this kind of information allows patients to establish a greater sense of control over their lives.

The relationship between you and your doctor is unique. Its success will depend on a variety of factors, including both your personalities and your philosophical approaches to health care. Because cancer is a chronic disease, the relationship will continue long after treatment ends. That's why it's so important that you feel you have the full support and cooperation of your physician.

The patient-doctor relationship is a two-way street. Be considerate of your doctor's hectic schedule and challenging workload, and try not to be unrealistic in your expectations.

As much as we might like to believe that doctors have all the answers, the reality is that they don't. If, like Dana, we insist on putting physicians on pedestals, we are bound to lose sight of them as human beings. Doctors aren't mind readers, and they aren't infallible. When something is bothering you, it's up to you to say so. As simplistic as that sounds, many of us have trouble remembering it.

If you find that the relationship with your doctor is becoming contaminated by angry feelings, arrange to discuss the matter candidly, either directly with your physician or with one of his or her colleagues (such as the doctor who initially referred you). If you are unable to resolve your conflict, don't think twice about finding another physician who is more responsive to your needs.

Emotional Entanglements

Oncology wards are hardly anyone's idea of a place for romantic rendezvous. Nonetheless, some patients find themselves caught up in sexual fantasies involving one or more of the people on their medical team. (This is especially true of breast cancer patients because of the strong sexual identification of the female breast.) For most patients these feelings amount to nothing more than a harmless crush, but for others they can take a more ardent form. In either case, an emotional involvement can make breaking away from the hospital world all the more difficult.

Monica, a fifty-two-year-old psychotherapist, underwent a mastectomy six years ago. Three years later she was operated on for stomach cancer, a malignancy unrelated to her previous breast cancer. She had surgery to remove her stomach and spleen and was given an intensive schedule of chemotherapy and radiation. Her prognosis was poor; the doctors gave her a 5 percent chance of survival. But Monica wasn't buying into the bleak statistics. Today she is in remission and back at work in her private practice.

I didn't feel any of that anxiousness about going off treatment, like so many other survivors do. Instead, my problem was letting go of the relationship with my doctor.

When I first met the oncologist after my diagnosis for stomach cancer, he asked if there was anything he could do. I told him, "Yes! Don't look so damn sad when you talk to me!" I knew my prognosis wasn't great, but I didn't want to get a mindset. We ended up having a wonderful working relationship. He was very professional and understanding, and we did a lot of joking around as well. He never quoted me statistics, and he was never pessimistic or patronizing. He knew I was a psychotherapist and so he treated me like a colleague.

Several months into treatment I started fantasizing about him. When I did, I'd get very emotional about our relationship. Deep down, I knew I had to stop this crazy obsessing, but I just couldn't let go of it. Sometimes when I'd see him reality would kick in. I'd realize how we both had happy, stable marriages and that all this fantasizing was crazy. But then a few days later I'd find myself daydreaming about him all over again.

Once during an office visit he told me, rather offhandedly, that I was one of his favorite patients. I remember hearing that and then suddenly blurting out, "But I thought I was your favorite patient!" I couldn't believe the way I was behaving. I'd reacted just like a child. Fortunately he was very diplomatic. I think he could sense what was going on with me.

The last time I saw him for treatment he said, "Good news! You won't have to see me for another three months." Now usually that's the kind of news every patient wants to hear. But not me. I remember thinking, Oh my God. What do I do now? After that, I would spend hours dreaming up reasons to call him just to have an excuse to chat.

Lots of women — and more than a few men — find that relations with their doctors become entangled in a web of seemingly crazy and confusing emotions. The dynamics of the traditional patient-doctor relationship can lay the groundwork for this. Some patients gain comfort and reassurance from a paternalistic approach in which the doctor acts as an authority figure and the patient dutifully follows orders. But because of the intense emotions that accompany a diagnosis of cancer, the patient's respect for the doctor can develop into more intimate feelings.

Patients may also project romantic feelings onto doctors as a sort of coping mechanism. Fantasy is after all an excellent way of deflecting or blotting out fear and pain. And why not? As survivors like Monica admit, daydreaming about the doctor is certainly a lot more pleasant than worrying about all the "what ifs" of cancer. Julie Steckel points out that this is why the separation phase of the patient-doctor relationship can be particularly difficult for some women.

Women have a tendency to make more emotional connections in their relationships, and they don't like having them broken. Men, on the other hand, often use separation as a way of delineating and setting boundaries in relationships. If the doctor is a man, an abrupt separation with the patient may be the only way he knows how to say goodbye.

I think that having romantic fantasies about a doctor is quite normal. It's a function of our dependency needs in a time of crisis. Our first love is for our parents, and that kind of relationship is often duplicated in the patient-doctor relationship. Also, many women have romantic notions that are based in part on their fantasies of having a strong, protective lover, and that again ties in directly to aspects of the patient-doctor relationship.

Monica's training as a psychotherapist helped her analyze her feelings and, in turn, understand what motivated them.

I was able to rationalize what I was doing and keep it in perspective. I realized that in this relationship the doctor was more important to me than I was to him. I was putting my life into his hands in the fervent hope that he would save it. He had become my knight in a white coat. After I figured that out, I started asking myself what it was that was missing in my life, what I was getting out of this infatuation. I would essentially do a therapy number on myself and that would keep my emotions in check.

These insights allowed Monica to see how emotionally dependent she had become on her physician. But sometimes the dynamics are reversed. Linda's close relationship with her oncologist is an example. A forty-two-year-old computer consultant, Linda was eight years into remission on her initial diagnosis of leukemia when she began suffering from chronic flulike symptoms. She called her family doctor, who suggested she call her oncologist.

I had kept the same oncologist since my first diagnosis. He'd followed my progress and I'd made a point of staying in touch with him. We had a very amicable relationship throughout my illness and recovery, but now that I look back on it I realize that perhaps the relationship was too close. In a way I had become like a trophy to him — I was one of his success stories; I was a *survivor*.

When I told him I wasn't feeling so great he refused to believe it might have anything to do with a recurrence. I finally insisted that he examine me for a possible malignancy. The tests came back positive — I had cancer again. He was devastated — and I wasn't too happy about it either. I had clearly not made his day.

My respect for him really took a nose dive after that. I felt used. My best interests were obviously not in the forefront of his mind. I was mad as hell, and very confused as to what to do. He's a skilled physician, a well-respected oncologist. I wanted him to treat me for this recurrence. But I sure didn't want to be just another feather in his cap.

When doctors let their own emotions get in the way, patients like Linda understandably feel angry and helpless. But Linda wanted to maintain the relationship with her doctor. She knew, however, that before she could reenter treatment under his care she had to clear the air.

I didn't want things to be poisoned by these bad vibes between us. I felt I'd get too emotional if I had a face-to-face talk with him, so I wrote him a letter instead. I told him that I could sense his disappointment in me for getting a recurrence. I asked him to put himself in my shoes. How did he think *I* felt? I explained that I needed a doctor who would continue to be optimistic and encouraging even if things weren't looking great. I asked him pointblank: "Can you provide me with that — along with the chemo?" If not, I said, I would find an oncologist who would.

He called me a few days later. He sounded pained by what had happened and apologized for giving off those vibes. It was true, he said, "I was upset that you of all people should have a relapse. I've known you a long time, and damn it, the news really shook me up." He said he hoped I would forgive him and added, "I hope you'll give me another chance. I feel confident that together we can beat it." I hung up the phone and felt so relieved that I cried. That telephone call did more for me than any medicine could.

Through the simple act of writing a letter, Linda renegotiated her patient-doctor relationship. Pen and paper were the forum for communicating her feelings and regaining a sense of control over her life. Although Linda is facing another round with cancer, she tells me she still feels like a winner.

Noncompliance

Not every wrinkle in the patient-doctor relationship can be ironed out. Sometimes during cancer treatment a patient will disagree with "what the doctor ordered." For any number of reasons, the patient may elect not to go through with a particular diagnostic test, to ignore instructions on medication, or even to refuse treatment. Such noncompliance poses a serious threat to the patient-doctor relationship.

Noncompliance is, I believe, a crucial subject, yet it is one that is often overlooked in most books on cancer. I have strong personal feelings on it as well since noncompliance was a pivotal issue in my breaking bonds with the hospital.

When I was diagnosed with rhabdomyosarcoma at age seventeen, my oncologist informed me that I would receive a yearlong regimen of chemotherapy as well as six weeks of radiation treatment. Needless to say, it was a tough year. Once I reached the end of the prescribed treatment, my oncologist recommended one more year of chemotherapy. At first I was shocked by the news; then I got angry. I couldn't understand why, with my cancer in remission, he was telling me I had to go through yet another year. I explained how the past twelve months had completely wiped me out. He thought the additional treatment would ensure my long-term survival, but I was unconvinced that it was necessary and told him I needed to think it over.

A week later I informed him that I had made up my mind: no more chemotherapy. During that week I had investigated treatment options for my type of cancer, consulting with oncologists familiar with treatment protocols for rhabdomyosarcoma and checking with several cancer research institutes. I learned that for my particular case, evidence from the latest studies supported shortened treatment regimens. My parents, who had helped in my investigation, fully backed my decision.

My oncologist vehemently disagreed with me, but I held firm. I had half expected his reaction but hoped that rather than getting upset he would simply wish me luck and offer reassurance. Instead we parted in silence, and I found another oncologist for follow-ups.

Like most people, I was raised to believe that when it comes to one's health, the doctor knows best. Disagreeing with the physician is a direct violation of this precept. To be sure, oncologists are experts in waging war against cancer. But as a patient, you may have different ideas about what is in your best interest. Treatment decisions ultimately rest with you. Yet survivors who decide to become "conscientious objectors" in the fight against cancer often leave the hospital burdened with anger, anxiety, and guilt.

The reasons the patient-doctor relationship can break down over the issue of noncompliance are varied. Some patients simply don't know enough about the medications they are taking and so, out of fear or mistrust, they react defensively. Others have legitimate concerns about the short- or long-term effects of treatment. For still others, noncompliance is a reaction to feelings of helplessness. Defying the physician is their way of asserting control over a disease that has rendered them powerless. Julie Steckel adds:

Sometimes there's a legitimate reason for the patient to be angry at or disagree with the doctor, and sometimes it's just part of how the patient reacts to a life crisis. And then there is always the "kill the messenger" syndrome. Because the doctor is the one breaking the bad news and dishing out the disagreeable treatments, the patient will vent all his anger and blame onto the doctor.

Noncompliance is by no means a recommended course of action. But if you do disagree with your doctor, you should be aware of the consequences of your decision and take full responsibility for it. It's a choice that could literally mean the difference between life and death. If you and your physician have an unresolved conflict, do everything you can to straighten it out. If, like Linda, you are uncomfortable talking directly to your physician, put your concerns on paper, or ask another doctor or hospital staff member to intervene on your behalf.

Don't overlook the importance of being a well-informed patient. And don't be nervous about asking your doctor to explain decisions about your treatment, if only so you can better understand his or her viewpoint. Many patients think that if they question their physician in any way they run the risk of losing their doctor's support. Every now and then that does happen. But on the whole most physicians are quite adept at fielding questions and mediating dissent.

I know now that when I met with my oncologist to discuss my decision I should have asked a social worker or some other member of the hospital support staff to accompany me. If I had, the meeting might not have ended in mutual anger. As it was, I didn't allow him to understand the considerations that motivated my decision. I also think it would have helped if his own attitude had been different. I wish he had said something like "I understand your decision. It's not the decision I would have made, but I support it." That would have made the situation much easier for me to handle.

Regrettably, it took me fourteen years to resolve that conflict with my oncologist. With the insights gained from my involvement in Cancervive, as well as through the inevitable process of maturing, I came to understand the tangle of emotions that made our last meeting such an angry event. I had come to terms with many painful aspects of my cancer experience, but the episode with my former oncologist was one of the last pieces I needed to work through. I decided to make an appointment with him.

We met, and after a few minutes of polite conversation the subject turned to our last meeting. He told me how worried he had been over my decision — hence his anger — and I reiterated my reasons for not undergoing further treatment. We both agreed that this discussion should have taken place fourteen years before. This time, however, we parted with new-found respect for each other.

Checking the Facts
with Your Physician

In making your break from the hospital world, you're bound to feel apprehensive about what lies ahead. During treatment, the doctors were calling the shots. Now responsibility for your well-being has shifted back to you. Be as vigilant and as assertive as you can.

If you haven't already, do as Dr. Richard Steckel suggests and schedule a "debriefing" session with your physician. By knowing what to expect in the months and years ahead, you can avoid or alleviate much of the fear and uncertainty that may accompany you home from the hospital. Here's a checklist of suggestions to guide you through your debriefing session.

- *Organize your meeting.* Before you schedule an appointment with your doctor, draw up a list of any questions you want to ask. If you wish, bring a friend, relative, or even a tape recorder to the meeting. The presence of an outside witness reduces the chance that you will misinterpret or forget an important point of information. Also, having a friend or family member in attendance gives you psychological support.
- *Get the low-down on your diagnosis, treatment, and any possible late effects.* As years go by, you may lose track of important information concerning your case history. It may not seem very important to you to differentiate between stage 1 and stage 3 Hodgkin's disease, but it makes a big difference to a physician. Be sure to ask your doctor for a written description of your diagnosis as well as a review of the treatment you received, and store this information with your important personal records. Also, find out what late or long-term effects of treatment you might encounter. Get as much information as you can; it will help you feel more confident and in charge of your recovery.
- *Be sure to check out your checkup schedule.* One of the easiest ways to ease anxiety is by keeping up with follow-up exams. Now that your cancer is in remission, periodic follow-ups will become an essential part of your maintenance program. Don't treat them lightly.

The kind of follow-up program your doctor recommends will largely depend on your type and stage of cancer. Generally speaking, for the first year after treatment you will probably be asked back for checkup exams every three or four months. After that — and again, depending on the type of malignancy — checkups will be either once or twice a year. Be sure to ask about the kinds of tests you can expect during your checkups. It's also a good idea to keep a personal written record of all your follow-up appointments and tests. You might find that it helps to jot everything down in a special follow-up datebook or calendar.

• *Find out who has an open-door policy.* It is important to your emotional health as well as your physical well-being to know that you can keep in touch with a member of your health care team. But remember that your oncologist or primary-care physician may be too busy with other patients to see you as often as you'd like. If that's the case, ask your physician to refer you to someone more available.

• *Learn how to be wary, not worried.* Part of the anxiety you feel after quitting treatment comes from knowing that responsibility for your health is now primarily up to you. It is normal to feel anxious. You may find that you get especially jumpy just before your follow-up visits. Even those sturdy individuals who never bothered to heed an ache or a pain before their cancer diagnosis suddenly find that the slightest twinge sends them flying to the doctor. We will deal with the issue of fear of recurrence in a later chapter, but it is important to mention here that this preoccupation with health is quite normal — even healthy — as long as it's not keeping you up nights.

3

Sizing Up the Emotional Aftermath

Healing is a matter of time, but it is sometimes also a matter of opportunity.

— Hippocrates

A FEW YEARS AGO I was asked to lead a workshop on peer support at a survivorship conference in Albuquerque, New Mexico. During a break I was approached by a tall man with a quiet, solitary demeanor. He introduced himself as Dennis and said that the day before had marked his first year free of non-Hodgkin's lymphoma. I congratulated him, and he smiled his thanks. But something in his eyes belied his smile. I asked if he wanted to talk after the workshop. We met for coffee, and he told me his story.

Dennis was a forty-one-year-old Vietnam veteran. Drafted at eighteen, he was badly wounded during a search-and-destroy mission outside Da Nang. For a few days following surgery, Dennis thought he was going to die. He didn't. Instead he recovered, was honorably discharged, and returned home to New Mexico.

After Dennis finished college, he married and settled down in Albuquerque, where he opened a sporting goods store. He put in fourteen-hour days and made the business a success. Life, he thought, was finally back to normal. But several years later Dennis was diagnosed with lymphoma, a cancer he suspects was caused by exposure to Agent Orange, the toxic defoliant used by U.S. forces in Vietnam.

I was certain that after Vietnam, nothing could come close to that experience. But I was wrong. It was hell all over again.

I was treated with chemotherapy at the local Veterans Administration hospital and got to know several other vets being treated for cancer. We'd spend a lot of the time swapping stories about 'Nam. Some of the guys did that, I think, as a way of getting their minds off cancer. It was safer for them to talk about that war than the one they were currently fighting. But to me it was all the same. I was right back in the trenches again, staring death in the face.

Actually, in some ways Vietnam was easier. At least you had furloughs, or you could get wasted and forget the war for a few hours. But cancer's different; it won't leave your head alone. Maybe that's because you're spending all your time and energy fighting something you can't even see. It's guerrilla warfare of a different kind. You wake up each day wondering, Am I going to win this one?

And I did — at least the first round. But after a few months, I started getting what my doctor called delayed stress reactions. It began with nightmares. I'd have a recurring dream that I was back at the VA for cancer treatment. I'd be all alone in the room, and then a group of Vietnamese would come in all dressed as doctors. That dream always ended the same way: this team of "doctors" would begin to strap me down on the table, and I'd wake up screaming.

The nights were affecting my days. I'd get into these angry moods and then snap at my employees. I started drinking heavily, and that made me even more antisocial. I knew I was in rocky shape, but I couldn't seem to make a move to get help for myself. No one could understand what I was going through. I was a survivor of two wars — and still a prisoner of both.

Dennis's story stirred up deep-seated feelings in me that I had trouble identifying at first. Though I'd never fought in Vietnam, I could empathize with the way he felt. But was it his war experience I connected with, or his cancer experience? As we talked, the line between the two seemed to blur. For survivors like Dennis and me, the similarities are striking.

The Psychological Wounds of War

"You have cancer."

With those three words, I suddenly found myself inducted into a battle I neither wanted nor understood. But I was not alone in the struggle: approximately one million Americans of all ages and backgrounds are impressed into it every year. And because cancer has a grim mystique all its own, it's quite unlike the fight against most other diseases.

Ambushed by aberrant cells within their bodies, cancer patients find themselves on unfamiliar terrain where the medical language is strange and disconcerting, the weapons debilitating and sometimes disfiguring. Dennis told me about how some of his fellow cancer patients at the VA hospital would sarcastically refer to treatment as "friendly fire." That reminded me of how Lisa and I used to swap "war stories" and compare our "battle scars" from surgery. For some patients, the fight against cancer is no more than a skirmish. For others, it's all-out war.

Once in remission, most survivors spend the immediate post-treatment period "licking their wounds" and assessing the physical damage done. But many discover that the emotional damage is not always as easy to recognize — or as accessible. In much the same way that soldiers return home with war still raging inside them, recovering cancer patients find they must struggle to come to terms with the full effect of their experience.

Until recently, Jesse, a survivor of acute nonlymphocytic leukemia, didn't understand why he was having such a hard time getting over his cancer experience, even though it was two years behind him. He talked about it with his support group.

My problem has its roots in my reaction to chemotherapy. As I got further along in the treatment protocol, I was increasingly freaked out by it. I mean, I knew the chemo was helping me, that without it I didn't have a chance. But even with sedation and antinausea medication, I'd get this very primitive panic-stricken reaction, like a trapped animal. As soon as I entered the treatment room I'd get sick to my stomach, and that would make me overreact even more. I'd do all those things you did as a child to manipulate yourself out of a bad situation. But nothing worked. I still had to sit there and have them run that I.V., and I knew all too well how and when it would kick in.

I'm a couple of years beyond that now, but my experience with chemotherapy still affects me. For instance, I have a lot of trouble being in a crowded room; anything like a busy restaurant or a packed elevator will set off feelings of panic. I may not show it, but inside I'm like a blender on high. I'll get all the signs of an anxiety attack: shortness of breath, rapid heartbeat, and nausea. My doctor says that it's common to have some delayed reaction to cancer treatment, but my case, he tells me, is extreme.

I know exactly how Jesse feels. Although I'm more than fifteen years past treatment, I still can't enter a hospital without experiencing strong physical reactions to my memories of cancer therapy. Whenever I enter an oncology clinic, I break into a cold sweat and my heart starts racing. The smell of alcohol pads and the sight of butterfly I.V.'s never fail to make me nauseous. Many survivors tell me they go through similar emotional responses, ranging from strong, persistent feelings of guilt and sadness to short bouts of insomnia and depression around the time of their follow-up exams. Survivors are especially prone to a rush of strong emotions before or on "anniversary" dates, such as the date they were diagnosed or when treatment ended.

But these reactions aren't unique to cancer survivors. Anyone who has endured a life-threatening or traumatic situation — an airplane crash, a violent crime, a devastating earthquake — is a likely candidate for a delayed stress disorder. Although many people appear to make a quick recovery from such a crisis, some experience long-lasting emotional reverberations that can take the form of recurring dreams, depression, phobias, substance abuse, and anxiety attacks. These symptoms may show up immediately following the trauma or develop seemingly out of the blue months or years later. Symptoms are often set off or made worse by physical reminders of the experience.

This delayed reaction to a traumatic event is called post-traumatic stress disorder (PTSD). But the name is only a new label for an old syndrome. During World War I, soldiers who exhibited psychological disturbances were said to be "shell-shocked" or suffering from battle fatigue. The Vietnam War ultimately brought the issue of post-traumatic stress disorder to national attention when reports focused on how the lives of many vets were disrupted — sometimes permanently — by the trauma of combat.

Dr. Richard Steckel of the Jonsson Cancer Center at UCLA comments on why cancer survivors are susceptible to PTSD:

People sometimes forget that the healing process from cancer can take a long time. Post-traumatic stress disorder should be viewed as an entirely normal and necessary coping mechanism. During the difficult phase of acute cancer care, you muster all your forces to pull through all the tests and treatments. You hold yourself together with that control. Once the treatment phase ends, that control is no longer needed, and any emotions you were suppressing will then rise to the surface.

It is important to accept these emotions and work through them so that eventually you can come to terms with what has happened. Most people recover from these delayed stress reactions given time, support, and counseling.

Without doubt, cancer does leave its dent in you. It could be that you feel changed, perhaps even transformed by the experience. You may discover, as I did, that who you are doesn't quite fit with who you used to be. As you begin to sort out what happened, that process is bound to generate strong emotions — rather like the aftershocks of an earthquake.

I've known survivors who have repressed or ignored those aftershocks, thinking that in time their unresolved emotions would take care of themselves. But the symptoms associated with PTSD don't vanish on their own. Instead they are likely to grow stronger and more insistent, until they start shaking up every aspect of your life.

How survivors go about reestablishing their emotional equilibrium after cancer is different for each person. It is important to remember, however, that although delayed stress reactions may not be avoidable, they are treatable. If cancer's aftershocks are rattling your recovery, grab hold of whatever therapeutic tools best help you cope with them.

One of the ways I faced up to my own delayed stress reactions was by keeping a journal. The process of writing helped me crystallize my thoughts and size up my emotions. Counseling helped too; through it I was able to take care of a lot of unfinished business.

As for my aversion to oncology clinics, I knew that was going to be a tougher nut to crack. I couldn't very well avoid hospitals without disrupting my follow-up schedule and ultimately jeopardizing my health. I tried different approaches, such as visualization and relaxation techniques, but nothing seemed to work. I did, however, develop two techniques of my own which have made a difference. For instance, I found it helps to have a friend or family member accompany me to appointments. I feel reassured by having someone along I can talk to when I feel anxious, or whose hand I can squeeze when I'm especially edgy. Also, I've learned how to "condition" myself by repeating in my mind during my appointments that I'm there only as a visitor, not as a patient. As a result, the oncology clinic is a much less threatening environment for me now.

Although visualization didn't work for me, Jesse says it has helped him with his phobia of crowded spaces.

I had a hard time accepting that I couldn't totally control my anxiety attacks. I really believed it was something I should be able to handle on my own. But I wasn't getting any better, and it was really upsetting me. I tried doing some guided visualizations that I read about in a book my therapist mentioned. Some days this helps a lot, but there are other times when nothing I do seems to help. My therapist referred me to a psychiatrist, who prescribed anti-anxiety medication. So now my approach is sort of half and half — which seems to do the trick. I do what I can through my own methods, and what I can't handle I leave to pharmacology.

Dennis had a more difficult time climbing out of the depression created by post-traumatic stress.

I don't remember having any real trouble adapting back to life after Vietnam. My therapist says the stress was there all along; I had just suppressed it. Then I got cancer, and I think that's what ultimately triggered a lot of long-buried memories. But even during treatment I wasn't doing anything to deal with the way I felt. Like in Vietnam, I thought I had to push those emotions aside and concentrate on making it out alive.

When I started drinking and getting depressed, one of the last things I wanted to do was see a doctor. I knew I needed help, but I was also fighting it. My wife couldn't stand living with me, though. She finally told me to get help or get out. Actually, she wasn't as ruthless as that. But she made sure I got help and pointed me in the right direction.

My psychologist treated me with hypnotherapy, and that brought a lot of stuff to the surface that I might not otherwise have faced. A doctor also prescribed medication to help control my mood swings. I'm not really into group therapy, but every now and then I'll drop by a vet support center just to touch base with some of the guys.

When I last talked to Dennis, he was in great spirits. He'd opened a second sporting goods store and was on his way to Hawaii with his wife to celebrate their tenth wedding anniversary. They were also celebrating Dennis's fifth year of remission.

"I don't fool myself anymore," Dennis told me. "I know I could have a relapse tomorrow. But something tells me I've fought all the battles I have to fight. I've earned my peace of mind. And I'll be damned if I'm not going to enjoy every minute of it."

Strategies for Adapting to Life After Cancer

Whether you realize it or not, cancer strikes at the very center of your identity. The post-treatment period is a time of reassessment, of trying to fit pieces of your old life into a new way of living. But absorbing the full force of these changes can take time. Coping strategies such as denial may work during the acute phase of cancer, but coping is by definition a short-term solution. As time passes you begin the lifelong process of distilling your reactions to cancer, as well as to any permanent changes it has caused. Perhaps without being aware of it, you'll formulate a long-term strategy for dealing with this new aspect of who you are. Survivors generally adopt one of three approaches:

- *Denial:* When survivors choose to disassociate themselves completely from the disease. They may even deny they ever had cancer.
- *Involvement:* When survivors see their cancer as a profound life-changing experience and then make it the centerpiece of their lives.
- *Acceptance:* When survivors find ways to accept what has happened, put it in perspective, and integrate the experience into their lives.

Is one strategy more effective than the others? Only you can decide which works best for you. But a word of warning: the first two approaches have inherent drawbacks.

DENIAL: WHEN THE ESCAPE HATCH BECOMES A TRAP

Many of us have felt the sting of cancer's stigma during diagnosis and treatment. The disease set us apart and swept us into "that other place," what Susan Sontag in her book *Illness as Metaphor* calls the "night-side of life." When patients leave the hospital, it makes sense that one of the first things they want to do is forget that cancer was ever a part of their lives.

That's understandable, and in the short run perfectly acceptable. Denial is a common way of coping with a threatening situation. It's the mind's way of protecting us from emotional overload. Denial allows us to absorb painful or stressful information in tolerable doses so that we can continue to function at a relatively normal pace. Virtually every cancer patient uses a certain amount of denial in dealing with the news of diagnosis ("It can't be true! This isn't happening to me!"). As a coping strategy, denial helps us push aside fear and replace it with hope and determination, the kind of emotions that enable us to mobilize for the fight against cancer.

Social worker Julie Steckel points out that survivors also use denial as a way of getting through the post-convalescent period.

Cancer patients don't necessarily stop denying just because treatment has stopped. For many people, cancer has forced them to let go of that sense of immortality we all unconsciously cling to. So the first part of the post-treatment phase may be one of total denial because of this lost view of mortality. Others must learn how to adjust to the loss of a body part and the image of who they used to be. Some patients have told me that their cancer experience was as traumatic as losing a loved one. All these losses require a time of mourning, a process of grieving.

This process usually begins with shock and disbelief — the initial reactions to a cancer diagnosis — and then continues on to include (in no set order) denial, anger, depression, and finally acceptance. It's going to be difficult for you to get to the acceptance stage if you miss or get stuck in any of the previous stages. Survivors should understand that denial is one part of that process, a necessary part of the progression toward healing. That process takes time; it can't be rushed. In short, some denial is healthy, as long as it doesn't sabotage the healing process.

It is understandable to want to avoid the pain of loss, and the most convenient way of doing that is to deny it ever happened. But there is a limit to what this strategy can accomplish. Denial offers a reprieve from reality, but the cost of that reprieve can be high.

That was the message of Claudia's story. The twenty-three-year-old graduate student spent three years in treatment following a diagnosis at age twelve of acute lymphatic leukemia. Denial became her modus operandi as a survivor.

About a year after I'd finished treatment I returned to the hospital for a checkup. One of the nurses spotted me and asked, "Hey, didn't I used to see you around here? Weren't you one of the kids we treated for leukemia?" I remember shooting her a look that said, Honey, you've got the wrong person. She persisted until I finally said, "Listen, I have no idea what you are talking about."

That was my way of dealing with cancer. I pretended it never happened. In my mind it was over and done with — and better forgotten. I thought that it simply had no bearing on who I was. Besides, the last thing I wanted was to be known as a cancer survivor. A lot of people still view it as a strike against you.

Claudia thought she had tossed her cancer experience to the wind. But years later, she says, it came flying back at her like a boomerang.

It happened the summer I graduated from high school. One day I was house-sitting for a doctor friend of the family when I started paging through a pile of her magazines. I ran across what looked like an intriguing article on cancer in a medical journal. Now cancer articles don't faze me. I know some survivors are phobic about the subject, but for me that was never a problem. The piece was a debate about whether or not the five-year survival period is an accurate indicator of a cancer cure. Several of the doctors in this article argued that the figure was a bogus statistic, that five years is no guarantee that a patient is cured.

As I read, my hands began to tremble and my heart started pounding. I remember getting this overwhelming rush of emotion, and then I felt like I couldn't breathe. Suddenly I hurled the magazine across the room and started screaming and crying. I mean I really fell apart. Somehow I managed to call my mother, and she came and got me. She couldn't believe the state I was in. I couldn't believe it either. I reacted this way even though my doctors had told me time and again that I was cured, and that the survival rate for my kind of cancer was very high.

I'm not sure what happened that day — or why. It was as if something inside me had given way. I'd finished treatment when I was fifteen, but it had taken me more than four years to come to terms with how my illness had devastated me emotionally.

Claudia believed she could go forward with her life by making a conscious effort to forget about cancer. But like Dennis, she found out how tenacious the emotions of unfinished grief can be. What began as Claudia's escape route from grief became a trap ensnarling her in the very emotions she sought to avoid.

One of the more dangerous aspects of denial is that it can allow you to "fall between the cracks" of the medical support system. In other words, by choosing to deny your cancer history you will inevitably lose sight of the importance of follow-up visits.

Ernest R. Katz is director of psychosocial and behavioral sciences at the Jonathan Jacques Children's Cancer Center in Long Beach, California. He believes that survivors who depend too heavily on denial are most likely to retreat from any identification with the disease. "Their attitude is, 'I'm tired of being different. I just want to melt back into the crowd.' That attitude is understandable, but it can also be dangerous to a survivor's physical health."

Such an approach is especially dangerous, says Dr. Katz, if recovered patients move to new communities and then decide to "forget" about their cancer history.

Sometimes if a survivor doesn't have any noticeable giveaway, such as a scar or other physical alteration caused by cancer, he might be tempted to "overlook" telling a new doctor about his cancer history. This can be a major problem for both the doctor and the patient since doctors make decisions about a patient's health based in part on the medical history. That is why it's so important for survivors to recognize and remember their cancer history, and realize that they will need follow-up care for the rest of their lives. Cancer's stigma is still the major underlying reason why many people continue to fall through the cracks, and we have to work at changing that.

Although selective denial is a valid method of coping with the immediate crisis of cancer, you should be aware of how dangerous it can be in the long run. When you let denial interfere with your physical health or affect your emotional equilibrium, this seemingly harmless strategy can become a very real threat to your well-being.

INVOLVEMENT: WATCH OUT FOR BURNOUT

Instead of turning their backs on cancer, some people throw themselves headlong into a whirl of cancer-related activities. They join nonprofit organizations, sign up for volunteer work, start self-help groups, or find some other way to connect to the topic of cancer. These survivors emerge from the experience with the strong desire to "give something back." Because cancer has rekindled their appreciation of life, they are eager to share their insights and give of themselves to others.

Christine Perkins is a psychotherapist who serves as Cancervive's director of social services in Los Angeles. She began internship work with cancer hospice patients eleven years ago after surviving a bout with uterine cancer. We recently talked about what motivated her involvement in cancer-related work.

I think that once you've survived a life-threatening illness there's a great sense of obligation, maybe even guilt. You've been given a second chance, and you're not sure why. It leaves you with the gnawing feeling that you should do something worthwhile with it. Through my involvement in both hospice work and Cancervive, I feel like I'm having a direct impact. It's my contribution, helping those who are going through what I went through.

I find that it's therapeutic as well. It has helped me work through some of my own fear and feelings of vulnerability. I've also learned a lot more about myself. As a survivor, I've got more to give now, more to share, on both a professional and personal level. And if survivors don't take responsibility, who will?

People who become involved in cancer-related activities are employing a useful adaptive technique that helps them handle the tangle of emotions which the disease dropped in their laps. By dedicating themselves to the cause of helping others with cancer, they gain a new sense of self-worth and accomplishment.

It is possible to go overboard, however. Too much involvement can lead to preoccupation. You can become so wrapped up attending.to the needs of others that your own needs are shunted to the wayside. Before you know it, you're overwhelmed and exhausted, and that's bad news for your immune system.

You may have, perhaps unconsciously, made a full-time career out of cancer. But if you insist on allowing it to take center stage, you should realize that other aspects of your life — family, friends, job — are going to be affected. Keep in mind that involvement is the flip side of denial. Instead of running away from the issue, you've jumped into the midst of it and gathered it around you like a blanket. Like denial, involvement can be an effective strategy for coping — as long as it doesn't become a permanent one.

Phyllis is one survivor who feels she has crossed the line into preoccupation. The divorced mother of three underwent a mastectomy six years ago. Following her operation, Phyllis went looking for emotional support in the suburb she lived in outside Seattle. To her surprise, no mastectomy support groups existed. She decided to organize one.

Anger was my initial motivating force. I was so pissed off that no one — including the hospital staff and administrators — could conceive that mastectomy patients might actually need a support group. I'll tell you, starting that group gave me back a sense of control over my life. It was liberating in so many ways. With every woman I encountered, I learned something new about myself. Also, through the group I was finally able to get rid of my anger, accept my cancer, and see it as a positive force in my life.

Sometimes, though, I feel as if this organization is engulfing me. I'm not trying to earn karma points or anything, but it's as if the support group has turned into my life's mission; I have *become* the organization. There are times when I'm not sure where my life begins and the group ends. Cancer has become such a large part of my life that I'm not doing a lot of the things I would otherwise do if I had the time. For instance, I can't remember the last time I took a vacation with my kids. I don't date as much as I'd like, and that bothers me too. Then again, I don't have the time and energy to do much dating. Sometimes I wonder if I'm using my support group to avoid other things.

Nora is another survivor who has involved herself in cancer-related activities as a means of coming to terms with her experience.

Lots of survivors tend to deny their cancer, but not me. I've done just the opposite. Since I beat stomach cancer two years ago, I've kept cancer right there in front of me all the time. I'm very active in a local nonprofit cancer education organization. In my private practice as a social worker I spend much of my time working with cancer patients. I also run a couple of small support groups.

Confronting this disease over and over again has helped me deal with a lot of personal issues. I find that my involvement reinforces the view I now have of myself as a survivor. But it has also created a few problems. It seems my missionary zeal is messing up my home life. For instance, my family and I recently had a big blowup. My husband and daughter told me that they didn't want cancer in their lives anymore. They said they were tired of hearing about cancer all the time, that I can't let twenty minutes go by without bringing up the subject. They'd just had it.

At first I was upset and defensive. I thought, How can they be that way? It's so unfair! But after I simmered down I realized that their needs were just as legitimate as mine. I *was* being obsessive about cancer, and they had reached a saturation point. We worked out a compromise. I've cut back on some of my activities, and they have promised not to give me grief on the things I need to do.

The approaches adopted by Claudia, Phyllis, and Nora parallel my own attempts at fitting in again after cancer. In the years since treatment I've used the strategies of both denial and involvement veering into preoccupation. For the first decade after my battle with cancer, denial served as my shield against rejection as well as protection from the psychological consequences of the experience. I adopted it not so much as a conscious choice, but rather as a reflex action. I eventually learned, however, in much the same way Claudia did, that denial is a temporary solution at best.

The chief reason many survivors adopt denial is that they cannot fully process what has happened. Cancer catches us off guard, and we plane our way through treatment on a layer of fear and apprehension. For months or even years we live a sort of wary, static existence. We finally emerge at the other end of treatment, only to be plunked down in the middle of an emotional nowhere land. No support system is waiting for us at the end of the line. Because we were so focused on the fight, most of us never fully anticipate the effect the illness will have on the rest of our lives. We don't even know how or where to begin making sense of it all.

Our first instinct, therefore, is to distance ourselves from the experience in an attempt to be "normal" again as fast as we can. And if that means avoiding cancer's residual emotions, so be it.

It wasn't until I started Cancervive that I realized how much I needed to understand the past and integrate its meaning into the present. The organization gave me the perfect excuse for shifting tactics. Like Phyllis, I charged into a long phase of preoccupation. By the end of my second year with Cancervive I'd reached burnout. As with Nora, my family was instrumental in calling my attention to my overinvolvement. With their help I came to see that I needed to formulate a more balanced approach. One of the ways I did this was by pulling back and allowing other people to take on some of the responsibility for running Cancervive. For instance, as much as I enjoyed one-on-one peer counseling, I also found it emotionally draining. I realized that if I was going to continue working effectively for the organization, I needed to establish some emotional distance from it. By curtailing my involvement in counseling I felt less stressed out and more focused. After swinging from denial to preoccupation, I'd finally reached a level of acceptance, a psychological centering, a comfortable middle ground.

It is essential that you find a way of righting your world after cancer has turned it upside down. But it is just as important to avoid extremes while you are making that adjustment. Full recovery depends not only on how well you manage the physical healing, but your own psychological recuperation as well. Acceptance of your cancer experience involves a continual appraisal of its meaning as it relates to every aspect of your life. You're bound to uncover several layers of emotions in the process. Let it happen. Work through them. Give yourself a chance to heal.

By finding the way to acceptance of your cancer you will be better able to glean from it its positive aspects. And there *are* positive aspects. I'm much stronger and more in touch with myself as a result of my acceptance of cancer. That's why seeking a source of support early on in your recovery is so important. If you wait, as I did, you run the risk of becoming entrenched in unresolved emotions, and when that happens you are blocked from reaching a state of peace within yourself. Cancer will remain the dark cloud that shadows you through life. With the help of private counseling or a support group, you have the opportunity to shake your fist at that cloud and even drive it away.

A Fuller Sense of Life

"There is a time of departure," the playwright Tennessee Williams once wrote, "even when there's no certain place to go." Without knowing precisely how or when it happened, most survivors realize that although they never left town their cancer experience has taken them on an amazing journey. When we look in the mirror we may see our faces as unchanged, but the persons they belong to have undergone a spiritual metamorphosis. We have shed our old skins. Now we must assess who we've become and where we're headed.

If that sounds intimidating, don't worry — it's not. On the contrary, it's time to start celebrating the good things we have gained from the experience: a whittling away of the inessential in life, heightened appreciation of family and friends, new insights into the depths of our spiritual strength, physical resiliency, and courage.

For all his troublesome reactions to chemotherapy, Jesse now recognizes how cancer served as a catalyst for personal growth.

Going through cancer was a painful experience, but it was also a learning experience. I've gained so much and changed in so many ways. In those two years I acquired insights that most people take a lifetime to realize. I guess you could call it wisdom, except most people are usually old and gray by the time they've accumulated it. Me? I've got a lifetime to enjoy it.

A battle with cancer strips life down to the bare essentials, and our values and priorities are often rearranged in the process. In a relatively short time we become filled with new and sometimes profound insights about ourselves and those around us. We view the world more clearly and feel it more intensely. Life is enriched simply by the awareness of its preciousness.

Many survivors come away from cancer determined to make life a bracing adventure — nothing less. They find themselves reinventing who they are, rethinking their lives, and plunging into activities they never before dreamed of doing. Nora observes:

Cancer has made me much more of a risk-taker. Before my diagnosis I was always one of those middle-of-the-roaders. You'd never catch me rocking the boat. Well, that's completely changed. In fact, now I go out of my way to look for challenges. Three weeks after I finished treatment, I slapped a bandage over my Hickman catheter and went parachuting. I would never have had the courage to do something like that before. And that's just the small stuff. I also became involved in lobbying efforts in behalf of a state bill regulating the disposal of toxic material. I feel that with whatever time I've got here, I want to agitate and make as many changes as possible. I want to make a difference. I wake up every morning thinking about all the possibilities. Life is there for the taking, and I plan to grab as much as I can.

Since the day her denial gave way, Claudia has invested much time and energy in reconciling herself to her cancer experience. It has, she says, provided her with unexpected dividends:

After three years of treatment, I left the hospital feeling as if I was floating away from the dock without any oars. I guess you could say I just bobbed along until a storm capsized me.

I started psychotherapy some time ago, and that's helped me resolve a lot of the feelings I'd stuffed away. Through a hospital social worker I found out about Cancervive, and I've been attending one of their support groups. I feel like I've uncovered a whole new part of myself. I don't feel ashamed anymore of having had cancer. In fact, people think I'm crazy when I talk about my cancer as being a *gift*. I'm beginning to understand how in many ways cancer was my upbringing, my education. It was the way I learned how to relate to the world. And it has everything to do with who I am today.

In the school of life, cancer survivors feel as if they've just completed an accelerated course — not that anyone, given the choice, would sign up for that course again. But for those fortunate enough to have gained a new perspective, the lessons learned are as precious as life itself.

Frances Feldman, professor emeritus at the University of Southern California's School of Social Work, shared with me one survivor's eloquent observation: "You have never lived until you have almost died, and for those who fight for it, life has a flavor the protected will never know."

4

Moving Beyond the Fear of Recurrence: Planning for the Future

CANCER HAS a strange way of playing havoc with one's sense of time. During the period of my diagnosis and treatment I remember feeling as if my life had abruptly come to a standstill, my horizons collapsing around the focal point of cancer. The clock and the calendar continued to proceed at their methodical pace, but I hung suspended in a sort of timeless limbo. There was no past, no future. There was just me, the disease, and the goal of getting through treatment.

Once past the experience, I found my perception of time changed yet again. I was now acutely aware of the time frame bracketing my existence. My plans for the future had to be retailored around a renewed sense of purpose, a need to make every minute count. Other survivors have shared similar impressions with me. "It's as if I can now physically feel the change of seasons, the melting of one day into the next," one woman remarked. "Cancer forced me to confront the fact that I don't have forever. Time is no longer a neutral part of my existence. I can't treat it casually anymore."

Her words reflect the urgency with which virtually every survivor approaches life. Once in remission, we settle into a cautious coexistence with cancer. Life's precariousness is all too tangible, and we aren't so cavalier anymore about what tomorrow may bring. But that acute awareness of time brings with it an underlying sense of vulnerability and persistent rumblings of anxiety. The only certainty, we now know, is uncertainty.

One of the challenges we as survivors face is living with that heightened sense of ambiguity, of pushing beyond fear and getting on with life. But that's not always easy to do. For survivors like Renée, forty-three, fear of the future is a major stumbling block to moving ahead.

Renée was treated for uterine cancer three years ago. Since then her doctors have seen no signs of recurrence; they say she's disease-free. But Renée says she continues to suffer from a kind of phantom illness: fear of recurrence.

After my surgery I thought everything would be okay, that I'd pick myself up, dust myself off, and go on from there. But it hasn't turned out that way. Surgery left me with a lot of complications. On top of that, I decided to call it quits with my husband. But the hardest part has been living with the fear of recurrence.

I've been in remission for more than three years now, and yet a day doesn't pass that I don't think about getting cancer again. I try to put it out of my head as quickly as I can, but some days those thoughts won't leave me alone. When that fear locks on to me, I just seem to shut down emotionally. To compensate, I go at everything with a frenzy. I throw myself into living moment to moment so that I don't have to think about the future. Whenever checkup time rolls around I become a real basket case. I mean, how do you turn that kind of fear off?

For the last six years I've worked as a nutritionist at a large hospital. I have all the credentials and experience to set myself up in private practice, but I honestly don't feel I have the motivation to do it. It's so hard to plan a career when you don't really believe you'll be around for it. I can't picture myself getting old. In fact, I have a hard time seeing beyond tomorrow. I'm even afraid to start up new relationships. In my past life — that's how I refer to my life before cancer — I was fairly confident about where my life was headed. But these days I feel rudderless.

Living Under the Sword

Fear of recurrence, even for long-term survivors like myself, is the most unsettling aspect of life after cancer. For months, even years after treatment, you may find yourself teetering between the relief and exhilaration of remission and the haunting fear of a recurrence or a secondary cancer. It's a tough high-wire act, freighted with enough anxiety and doubt to throw anyone off balance. This state of apprehension, dubbed the Damocles syndrome by doctors, is one of the most frustrating obstacles cancer survivors face when it comes to getting their lives back on track.

Perhaps you know the story of Damocles. Greek mythology records that he was a courtier of King Dionysius, ruler of the ancient city of Syracuse. According to legend, Damocles was forever flattering his sovereign, impressed by the luxurious and secure life the old king appeared to lead. One day Dionysius decided to teach his courtier a lesson. He thought it time Damocles realized that however carefree and idyllic a sovereign's life might appear, it is never free of danger.

The following day, Damocles received an invitation to a royal dinner at the palace. He was delighted; such a perk was exactly what he'd been waiting for. That night Damocles found himself seated in the king's place, as the guest of honor. Ready to partake of the sumptuous banquet, he happened to look up. There above his head hung a large sword suspended from a single thread. Legend doesn't record whether Damocles stayed for dessert.

For survivors like Renée, remission in many ways resembles

that dinner for Damocles. It's hard to focus on the future when the possibility of a relapse seems to hang so perilously close. Cancer is no longer an immediate threat, but rather a cruel tease.

Some people are successful at managing their fear of recurrence. They refuse to be intimidated by uncertainty; it's just not their style. These survivors prefer to adopt an attitude of cautious optimism. They fully expect to survive cancer and live accordingly.

Others choose selective denial as their means of adjusting. A few go so far as to believe that because they've already had cancer, they are now immune from future malignancies. Using denial to blot out bleak statistics or unfounded fear is harmless, even healthy, as long as you don't let it obscure common sense. Should you find yourself "forgetting" about follow-up exams because you feel invulnerable to cancer, you've let your denial reach the danger level.

In general, however, most survivors find that fear of recurrence is an unwanted yet inescapable reality. As one survivor said, "It's sort of like having Muzak playing ever so softly in your head all the time. After a while you get used to it, but you never forget it's there."

You may notice that certain events tend to crank up the decibel level — when you're scheduled for a doctor's appointment or follow-up exam, for example, or at the appearance of some new and disconcerting physical symptom. "Anniversary dates" such as the day your cancer was diagnosed or the date you were declared in remission also become emotional red flags.

Pamela, a concert violinist, is a Cancervive member whose fear of recurrence ties in to her sense of physical well-being.

Since my breast cancer two years ago, pain has become my leitmotif. A sharp pain in my left breast was my very first clue to having cancer, even before I felt a lump. I had always heard that if it hurt, it wasn't cancer. The painless bumps and lumps were the dangerous ones, or so I thought. I'd long had a problem with benign cysts anyway, so I really didn't think it was any big deal.

But it was a big deal; it was malignant. I was lucky, though. Treatment worked, and I had no long-term effects to speak of — except one. Even though I'm physically recovered, I'm now saddled with this terrible phobia of pain. Whenever I get a headache I'll immediately think, Oh, great. I've got brain cancer. If my shoulder hurts, I naturally assume it's bone metastasis. My husband calls me a hyper-hypochondriac. I'm sure my doctor is about ready to lobotomize me — I'm always calling him to report what I'm convinced are the telltale signs of recurrence. He says I need to learn to let go of that fear. "Take time out to smell the roses, Pam," he tells me. That's easy for him to say. Hell, I'm having trouble even finding them.

One of the first facts survivors learn to live with is that, like heart disease or diabetes, cancer is a chronic condition. But that doesn't mean it can't be controlled and in many cases cured. In fact, cancer is considered to be the most treatable of chronic diseases. But no remission comes with a money-back guarantee, and cancer can be a poor loser. Just when you think you've won the fight the disease may pop up again, demanding another round in the ring.

That is why recovered cancer patients tend to live by one key word: surveillance. Many survivors tell me they are much more tuned in to their bodies since their cancer. But as Pamela knows, sometimes the surveillance act can get the better of you. It's as if, she says, "a hyperactive little sentinel has set up watch in a corner of my mind. Any cough or ache, any bump or bruise is all it takes for him to start screaming: '*Recurrence! Recurrence!*'" With a little work and lots of time, you'll eventually succeed at turning down the volume on this noisy alarm system.

But tuning it out altogether isn't quite so simple because at the heart of fear of recurrence lies our greatest, most unresolved fear: that of death and dying. Of course we also worry about the other elements of a relapse: going through treatment, suffering its side effects, having to put our lives back on hold. We wonder where we'll get the strength and will power to go through it all again. Yet deep down inside we know that if it comes to that, we can handle the physical battle. But what about the metaphysical one? Can we outwit death a second time? That's the real dilemma, the ultimate unknown. And it is the primary cause of our fear.

During the writing of this book I felt the long cold fingers of that fear for the first time in fifteen years. I developed an infection in my leg and was subsequently hospitalized for several days. During my stay I decided to go ahead with my yearly follow-up exam. I spoke with the hospital's director of oncology and the next day underwent the usual battery of tests: computerized tomography (CT) scans, magnetic resonance imaging (MRI), X rays, blood work.

Two days later I learned that one of the CT scans had picked up a suspiciously enlarged lymph node in my pelvic area. I knew something was terribly wrong when I was asked to submit to still more procedures — including a needle biopsy. These tests, however, proved inconclusive. After discussing my options with the surgeon, I decided to wait four weeks and then repeat the scan. If the lymph node grew in size, I'd have no choice but to undergo surgery.

I don't remember ever feeling so frightened, so helpless. Even during my initial bout with cancer I had never been so filled with terror. At the time, anger was my dominant emotion; I didn't know enough to be frightened. I knew better now, and I understood all too well what I was up against. Fear numbed and disoriented me, disturbed my sleep and concentration. Each day brought vivid flashbacks of my earlier experience with cancer. Could I go through that again? And what were my chances of beating it a second time?

Even though I was a long-term cancer survivor, this kind

of raw, elemental fear was new to me. Following my initial treatment, I was never really troubled by any worries about recurrence. I suppose I found it easier to ignore the possibilities. Then again, I live in California — earthquake country — and was used to living with uncertainty. I could spend my life huddled under a table waiting for the Big One to hit, or I could prepare as best I could for that eventuality and then go on about my business. Life after cancer, I thought, should be no different.

Now, as I lay under the massive CT scanner, my mind raced as the machine whirred and clicked. I thought about how insulated I'd become from the reality of being a cancer patient. Time had granted me distance from the experience but not, it seemed, immunity.

My doctor called me with the news that night: the abnormality was still visible. In fact, it had grown larger. He wanted me in for exploratory surgery within the week.

I wanted to wake up from this nightmare, but I didn't know how. I needed to think straight, to make decisions and formulate plans. The best antidote for my fear, I found, was to keep busy and constantly remind myself that cancer was only a possibility — not a certainty.

I awoke several hours after the operation to the rhythmic beeps of the monitors surrounding my hospital bed. Through my grogginess I could make out the blurry outlines of my husband and parents. They were smiling and giving me the thumbs-up sign. The surgery had proved negative; there was no sign of cancer.

Although that crisis is over, I find that I am still sorting through the emotional fallout it provoked. I now know, in a way I never had before, how powerful and disabling the fear of recurrence can be. But I also understand that this fear is one of the few things I am in a position to control. I know that if I don't, it will end up controlling me.

Fighting Fear

Fear is a misunderstood emotion. By itself it is not necessarily harmful or dangerous. Like stress, it acts as a warning signal; it's the body's way of alerting us to danger. It impels us to mobilize against the cause of our fear. In its own way, fear protects us.

That's its helpful side. Fear becomes harmful when it is denied or ignored, or when it is allowed to grow to such proportions that it overwhelms us.

"Fear of recurrence paralyzes some survivors and causes others to become preoccupied, frenetic, or even reckless," says Dr. Jordan Wilbur, chief of pediatric oncology at Children's Cancer Research Institute at the Pacific Presbyterian Medical Center in San Francisco. He observes that some survivors become so caught up in their fear that life becomes an intolerable waiting game, a kind of emotional stakeout.

One of the most frustrating things for me to see is survivors who have allowed the disease to dominate their thoughts to such an extent that it undermines their life. They may have won the battle against cancer on a physical level, but on an emotional level they've lost it.

When I see that going on, I'll try talking to the person. I'll say, "Listen, you had a disease that could have killed you, but it didn't. And now you're still letting it get to you. If you are going to take on the victim role, that's okay, if that's what you really want. But you should remember that it can become a habit — one that can be hard to break." For some of these patients it is very convenient to make cancer the scapegoat for everything that goes wrong. I think it's important that these patients recognize what they are doing to themselves.

Dr. Ernest Katz of the Jonathan Jacques Children's Cancer Center notes that adapting to the possibility of recurrence is a uniquely personal matter; every survivor handles it differently.

It depends on the individual's ability to come to terms with the initial cancer experience. Some people happen to be better than others at handling fear and uncertainty. I've seen some patients finish treatment who are really gung-ho about plunging back into the mainstream. They have somehow used their illness as a way to get their lives together.

Others find that their cancer took them out of the mainstream and left them there. It may be that it shut down opportunities and old goals. Some of these people allow themselves to get stuck in the cancer experience. As a consequence they approach life tentatively and often become bitter and depressed.

Few people have an easy time of coping with the unknown. As Dr. Katz points out, how you deal with the fear of recurrence largely depends on your attitude and the way you handle the problems life throws your way. You can either turn toward fear or away from it. Obviously, ignoring your fear isn't going to get you very far; denial serves to mask rather than mitigate a problem. But by acknowledging your fear you've taken the first step toward coming to grips with it. After that you can begin to map out a strategy for resolving it.

What strategy will work best for you? Some survivors have been able to modify the way they think about fear through visualization, meditation, relaxation techniques, therapy, and prayer. Others have gained a sense of control by altering their behavior — changing their diet and exercise habits, for instance, or adjusting their work schedules, or setting goals and planning for the future. One of these strategies may suit your needs — but then again, perhaps none of them will. There is no step-by-step recipe for quelling fear, and only you can know what method will work for you. To find an effective strategy you'll need to take stock of your unique strengths and abilities, then draw on your own inner resources. Try to determine what is most comfortable and workable for you.

For instance, your approach to problem solving may be analytical in nature; that is, you work best when you've had a chance to look at all the facts. The more you know, the better you feel. That was Pamela's way of dealing with her pain-related fear of recurrence.

I didn't like the feeling of being so paranoid about my health. I'd read in a book that time and a positive attitude would eventually take care of it. But how much time? How many years? I'm not that patient a person.

I've never been a big fan of all the New Age stuff, the miracles through meditation and macrobiotics routine. The way I usually deal with problems is to approach them cognitively — think them through, intellectualize them if you will. That's my way of mastering a situation. For me, knowledge is power. I needed to understand *why* I was letting every little twinge drive me up the wall.

I went back into private therapy. That gave me a chance to hash it out with an objective sounding board. I discovered that what I feared most was my own body. Before my cancer I'd never experienced any real illness or disability. I took my health for granted and naively expected my body would take care of itself. But with the cancer, I felt it had betrayed me. I didn't trust my body anymore; if it happened once, why shouldn't it happen again?

Well, of course, I know it can. I'm aware that I can't totally control everything that happens to me. But there are some things I can do. To start, I sat down with my doctor and asked him to tell me what I needed to know about recurrence, where it would most likely happen, the time frame, my chances, the whole routine. I don't know why I never thought of doing that before. I noticed that just talking it over with him helped me see how overblown my fear was, and that helped reduce its power over me.

I've taken other steps as well. My husband has always been much more health-conscious than me. He's also a better chef. Since all this happened he's been really marvelous about putting up with all my worrying. He took it upon himself to revamp our diet so that I'm eating only the foods I know are good for me — plenty of fresh fruits and vegetables and whole grains. From what I've read, they may even offer some protection against a recurrence. I've always found it difficult to exercise regularly because I travel so much of the year. But I've made a concerted effort to get back into a routine. My husband has taken on the role of personal trainer; he makes sure I stick to it.

Did all this make me less of a hypochondriac? Not exactly. I still get uptight over the odd ache or pain, although I find it's less of a problem. I just don't let myself obsess about it anymore. I'd rather spend that energy on something useful.

For survivors like Pamela, knowledge is a powerful tool against the fear of recurrence. Most people have an easier time coping with a problem once they have the full picture. When you don't know what to expect, your imagination tends to shift into overdrive, and that can fuel fear. Once you have a clear idea of what you can anticipate in the months and years ahead, the future will appear less ominous.

Pamela's approach also worked for me. By having some idea of what to expect if my surgery revealed cancer, I felt more in control of the situation. I also found it therapeutic to talk things over with family, friends, and other Cancervive members. Sharing my fears allowed me to release anxiety and put my feelings into perspective. What's more, I realized that a diagnosis of recurrence or secondary cancer didn't mean I was doomed. I count among my friends people who have survived more than one relapse. I know that recurrence doesn't mean certain death any more than an initial diagnosis does. This knowledge comforted me and kept fear from overpowering me.

Ironically, my recent false alarm not only triggered potent fears of recurrence but in the end allayed them as well. During that period I was put through what seemed like an interminable series of tests and procedures. None of them revealed cancer. My operation, as dreaded as it was, sounded the final "all clear" signal. And for now, that's what keeps the recurrence bogeyman at bay.

I ran into Renée a few months ago and was delighted to

hear she'd made a lot of progress. "I still catch myself getting depressed occasionally about all the 'what ifs,'" she told me. "But I have found a few strategies that seem to be working. I'm actually beginning to feel that maybe I'll survive after all."

I first met Renée over a year ago when she called the Cancervive office to find out more about the organization. I told her about an all-woman support group we ran and suggested she might like to attend. Here were Renée's impressions:

I went to a meeting and was relieved to see that I wasn't the only person whose life seemed to be thrown off track by fears of recurrence. I had tried talking over my fears with my family and one or two close friends, but they never knew what to say to me. I think more than anything it made them uneasy. It was just the opposite of that in the support group. I listened to other people — some of them seemed to be having a harder time than I was — and it dawned on me that I didn't need to be so entrenched in fear. I saw what it had done to one or two of the women in my group and I thought, *Am I going to let that happen to me?*

I got a lot out of that meeting. It does help to talk with people who know the ropes, so to speak, who have been through it themselves. But the trouble was, I just wasn't completely comfortable in a support group. I could never seem to really open up and relax. I talked to the group facilitator and she gave me the name and phone number of another woman, someone who shared my concerns and has gone through a similar cancer experience.

I'm not a real extroverted person, so it took me a few weeks to get around to calling this woman. The facilitator had told her about me, so when I called she seemed happy to hear from me. We went out for coffee later that week and hit it off right away. In a lot of ways Joan is the exact opposite of me. But the facilitator was right, we do share a lot of the same survivor problems. Joan told me how fear of recurrence had all but paralyzed her after her successful treatment for stage 2 uterine cancer. Like me, she couldn't really make any plans for the future because as she said, it all seemed so useless. We also share a problem with money; neither of us seems to be able to save it. I mean, what's the point if you're not going to be around to spend it?

"So let's just kill ourselves now and get it over with," Joan will joke. She's like that. She cuts through a lot of the crap with her sarcasm and one-liners. Joan has done a lot of work on herself. She's a lot further along in being able to manage her anxiety than I am, so she gives me pointers. For example, she says that one of the ways she's been able to condition herself to the idea of saving money is by investing in short-term certificates of deposit. She started out investing in three-month CDs. When she got comfortable with that, she started extending them out to six months and then one year. She suggests I try it.

She also suggests I try saving money for something I can really look forward to, like a big shopping spree or a vacation somewhere exotic. That idea really appealed to me. So I've been putting away part of each paycheck for a trip to Europe next spring with my cousin. I know that most people wouldn't consider that an accomplishment, but it is for me. I figure if I can do that, I'll have made it over a big psychological hurdle. As Joan says, it's just a matter of putting yourself out there, taking chances, not letting fear hem you in.

I do feel as though I've made a lot of headway. I guess I needed to reach my psychological bottom first. After that there was no way to go but up. I was buying some travel books the other day, and it occurred to me that for the first time in my "new" life I was really feeling optimistic. Next summer will mark my fourth year of remission, and I can honestly say that it's finally beginning to feel like reality.

For most survivors, fear of recurrence recedes with time as the pressures and pleasures of daily life crowd that foreboding to the back of the mind. But because survivors must live with follow-ups and other less imposing reminders of their cancer, that fear is bound to well up from time to time. If it becomes chronic or begins to impair your ability to get on with your life, find a way to fight back. Don't let fear hold you hostage. You didn't survive cancer only to spend the rest of your life worrying about it.

Some people hold back from seeking help because, as one man told me, "It's *my* problem, in *my* head. I should be able to handle it." He's right — half right, anyway. Fear is all in your head, but that certainly doesn't mean it's entirely up to you to resolve it. If you are having trouble, there's no law that says you can't get help. That's what friends and family, therapists, and support groups are for.

If you find you can't fully conquer your fear, it's important to keep in mind that in time it will become a less intrusive part of your life. There may be times when you feel as if you are not making much progress, but remember that with each passing day your chances of long-term survival improve.

Charting the Future

One of the most frustrating aspects of fear of recurrence is the way it can overshadow your view of the future. Renée is just one of many survivors I know who have difficulty making plans because they lack confidence in their ability to fulfill them. They have lost their future orientation, and as a consequence they feel as though they are, in Renée's words, rudderless in a sea of uncertainty.

Twenty-two-year-old Melanie knows the feeling all too well. She was diagnosed with rhabdomyosarcoma at age five. Fortunately, her long and intensive treatment proved successful. But five years later she was diagnosed with a secondary tumor, a highly malignant radiation-induced osteosarcoma. Once again, Melanie beat the odds. Over the last fifteen years, however, she has endured more than forty operations as well as several rounds of radiation and chemotherapy. These battles have left their mark on her, physically and psychologically.

Because I was under treatment for so long and from such an early age, I feel as if I've lost a great deal of control and responsibility for my own life. I don't remember making any real decisions for myself while I was growing up; so many of them were made for me by my

parents and the doctors. It was as if my body didn't even belong to
me anymore.

Somehow I managed to get through school, even with all the in-
terruptions. I never enjoyed it much, though. It was so hard to fit
in. I always felt like people were judging or pitying me. There were
teachers who would give me good grades, no matter what kind of
work I did. I could never gauge how smart I really was. I knew all
this medical stuff, platelet counts and radiation doses, but that kind
of knowledge doesn't really help when you're supposed to be studying grammar and algebra.

In my last year of high school I became very sick with another
complication. After I got better I thought about going to college but
then never really pursued it. I've sort of drifted along ever since. I
still live with my parents and I work part-time as a receptionist.
People used to ask me what I wanted to do with my life, and I'd just
draw a blank. When I tried to focus on plans, I felt lost and helpless.
It's not that I was scared of a recurrence. I'd been through too much
for that to bother me. I was just afraid to think on my own. When
you've spent so many years fighting for your life and then that goal
is suddenly taken away, you're left with this vacuum at the center.
You keep wondering, Now what? How do I top that goal?

The future, so long on hold for young cancer patients like
Melanie, frequently becomes daunting new territory once
they have achieved remission. It now requires rescouting and
rethinking. During treatment a patient's view of the future
telescopes down to the goal of running the medical gauntlet
and emerging victorious. With remission, the future looms
back into view — and for some it's an ominous sight.

Like Melanie and Renée, you may have trouble extending
your view beyond the here and now. Cancer has lit the wick
on your sense of mortality. You may feel as if you're living on
borrowed time, and that investing in the future is futile.

As a consequence, you may find yourself adopting a "live
for today" approach to life. With the future so ambiguous, it's
much easier to live in the certainty of the moment, attempting to wring as much happiness as you can from each day.
But as important as it is to "seize the day," too much emphasis

on today can cause you to lose sight of tomorrow. What's wrong with that? Nothing much, if you don't mind drifting and bobbing your way through life.

In my view, to live without hopes and aspirations isn't really living at all. It's merely existing. As human beings we are the only creatures with the capacity to rise above the struggle for existence and create meaning and purpose in our lives. Unlike other species, we can look beyond today and influence what happens tomorrow. But having that ability and using it are two different things.

Since I began Cancervive, goal setting has grown to be an essential and invigorating part of my life. I can plot my own personal progress as well as that of the organization against my goals. During the writing of this book, for instance, I flew to Dallas to attend a fund-raiser celebrating the start of a new chapter of Cancervive. While on the trip I formulated plans to start another new chapter in New York and one other city within the next six months. Setting this goal provides me with a tangible challenge — and a sense of accomplishment once I've realized it. Each new chapter represents a milestone in my overall objective of expanding Cancervive into a national organization. It's a matter of looking down the road and then moving ahead one step at a time.

Paul, thirty-two, is another survivor who uses goals as a means of getting beyond the desire to dwell in the safety and security of the present. I've known Paul, a hospital administrator, for several years, and I've always enjoyed his irrepressible optimism and drive. He believes that it was his sense of purpose, his sheer determination, that helped pull him through his first bout of stage 3 Hodgkin's disease at age eighteen. Ten years later he had a relapse — but that didn't stop Paul.

I found that the easiest way to get through my initial treatment was to focus on short-term goals. My primary goal at the time of my ini-

tial diagnosis was to get into Princeton. I essentially wanted two
things out of life: a good education and a chance to play college
football. Make that three things: I also wanted to beat cancer.

I remained focused on those goals and I think they had a lot to
do with my bouncing back quickly after treatment. I was so busy
working toward making those plans a reality that I didn't have time
to worry about recurrence. Also, I really needed to prove to myself
and to everyone else that I wasn't a disabled person. I *had* to believe
that my goals were within my grasp — despite the fact that I'd had
cancer. So I really pushed myself, both academically and athleti-
cally. I went to Princeton, became an honors student, and made of-
fensive guard on the football team.

Nowadays I try not to think much about cancer. When I do, I use
those feelings to push myself along. I use that fear as a reminder
that even though I'm young, I don't have forever. If I do spend too
much time dwelling on the negative aspects of the disease, that's
when it gets the better of me. Part of the problem is that society sees
me — all survivors, really — as short-term players. And if we aren't
careful we start believing it ourselves. But I reject that view. I feel
like I'm cured, and my doctors think so too. Cancer is a part of
my history. And if you forget history, you're never going to learn
from it.

For Paul, working toward the future adds significance to
life. He thrives on the sense of accomplishment that comes
from setting high goals and then achieving them. "I hate not
knowing where I'm headed," he says. "I don't want to spend
my life feeling as if I'm wandering blindly down some dark
corridor."

Goals provide direction; they're steppingstones to the future. Your goals don't have to be colossal to be effective. You
may no longer have the physical energy to tackle major goals.
Sometimes getting through the day is the only goal you can
muster. While you are striving to take charge of your life,
keep your plans for the future modest and realistic.

Grace Christ, director of the department of social work at
New York's Memorial Sloan-Kettering Cancer Center, notes:

Setting short-term goals for yourself is really the easiest approach to dealing with the future. It gives you a sense of moving ahead. The best way to start is to focus on plans for next month. If that's too far for you to project, ask yourself why you think that is. You may want to pose the question "Will I still be around in a month?" Chances are you can answer it affirmatively. As you gain confidence, begin to extend your plans to include longer-term goals. The important thing is not to overwhelm yourself with impossible ambitions or unattainable objectives. They will only serve to discourage you.

Renée and her friend Joan used this approach to tackle their fears of recurrence and the future. But some survivors are more comfortable letting the future take care of itself. For Melanie, this approach isn't so much a choice as a need.

Here I am, seventeen years after my first diagnosis, and I feel as if I'm just starting out in life. I realize I have a lot of catching up to do. For instance, I'm just now getting my driver's license. I feel as though I need to do so much growing up before I can even think about what I want to do with my life.

The older brother of a friend of mine is a recovering alcoholic who attends Alcoholics Anonymous meetings. Their slogan is "One day at a time." I think that's an acceptable way to live. I mean, I don't discount the future. But I can't trust it either.

Still, I know that I just can't sit around waiting for the rest of my life to happen. I need to sort out my priorities. It's really up to me to get things moving.

Redefining Priorities and Retailoring Old Goals

Fear of recurrence is perhaps the strongest psychological restraint preventing survivors from moving forward with their lives, but it's not the only one. At support group meetings I frequently hear survivors talk about how cancer has rearranged their priorities, scrambled their plans, and shifted their outlook on life.

Life-threatening diseases are like that. They have a tendency to turn your values inside out. Money or power may not be as important to you as it once was; then again, perhaps it is more important now. Many survivors discover that cancer has left them with a better idea of what they want out of life. Whether it's fulfilling a career goal, realigning a lifestyle, striving for spiritual beliefs, or reaching out to other people, cancer is often the catalyst.

But cancer can create unforeseen obstacles as well as new insights. Sometimes you need to make compromises. In order to fit into your new life, old plans and goals may require retooling.

Paul, for instance, was forced to alter his career goals because of his illness.

Medical school is one of the few objectives cancer thwarted. Ever since I can remember I've wanted to be a pediatrician. During treatment it never occurred to me that my illness might affect what I'd want to do with the rest of my life. But when I applied to several grad schools they either denied me admission or wait-listed me — which I felt amounted to the same thing.

I needed to find out what was going on. I called a friend of my father's who was assistant dean at a well-known medical school. I asked him about my chances of being accepted. He told me that even though my academic and athletic background was impressive, his school wasn't willing to enroll someone with a cancer history. Their thinking was that a person with a history of serious illness probably wouldn't be suited to the rigors of medical school.

I hung up the phone feeling as if I'd been hit by a truck. I remember thinking, What *else* do I have to do to prove myself? Here I was, about to graduate with honors from Princeton. I'd played four years of collegiate football. I'd even been drafted by an NFL team! Who were they to tell me I couldn't handle the rigors of medical school? I figured that the only way to beat the system was to become a part of it. So I decided to go into hospital administration. Now I'm chief operating officer at a large hospital in San Francisco — and doctors are working for *me*.

Robert Louis Stevenson once wrote, "Life is not a matter of holding good cards, but of playing a poor hand well." As a survivor, you may sometimes feel as if society has stacked the deck against you. Your career goals, like Paul's, may have been thwarted, not necessarily by your own physical limitations, but because of discriminatory policies. Adjusting to the compromises cancer imposes requires flexibility and perseverance as well as a dash of courage. When you encounter hurdles, don't let them hang you up. Find a way over or around them. In 1982, athlete Jeff Blatnick was diagnosed with Hodgkin's disease. But Jeff wasn't about to let cancer interfere with his dream of entering the Olympics. Two years later he made it to the Olympic games in Los Angeles — and captured the gold medal for wrestling.

Dr. Jordan Wilbur points out that when it comes to creating a life plan, each of us has an important choice to make.

You can either play the victim, which means you are going to let circumstances control your fate, or you can accept the fact that you, like anyone else, will have problems to contend with in life. You can work with those problems, and whatever limitations they put on you, and still do what you want with your life. As simple as it sounds, it does help to focus on the good rather than the bad. Of course, a positive attitude isn't going to make all those problems vanish overnight. But it will give you the energy and inspiration you need to work at solving them.

When I met a survivor named Ken at a Cancervive meeting not long ago, I was touched by his determination and courage. Ken, thirty-eight, is a successful interior designer. At the time he was diagnosed with lymphoma three years ago, his illness forced him to set aside plans for a spectacular house he was building in New Mexico. Ken's treatment was effective, however, and before long he was back on track with his construction plans. But last year Ken experienced another setback when his lymphoma returned. Now in remission, Ken recently talked to me about how he's managed to persevere through it all.

After my initial diagnosis my doctor didn't tell me much. I had no idea what kind of cancer I was dealing with or what my chances were. So one day while I was in for treatment I sneaked a look at the pathology report, and then I did some research. I learned that the kind of lymphoma I had is considered virtually incurable and is notorious for recurrence. I was reeling from the news for days.

I needed something positive to grab hold of to keep me afloat. That's when I started focusing on my plans for the house. I carry around a photo in my wallet of this place I'm building in New Mexico. I have no plans to stop construction, even though I have a pretty fair chance of having other recurrences. I really believe that this house is what keeps me going.

I first made plans to move to Santa Fe five years ago. I was born and raised there, and it's where my parents live. It had always been in the back of my mind to go back and build a house in Santa Fe and put down roots. When I got cancer, that dream suddenly became all-important. I dangled it in front of myself like the proverbial carrot. All during chemotherapy I would distract myself by daydreaming about that house. I designed every room of it in my mind. It became my escape routine, my way of coping. I guess you could say it's the house that cancer built.

So far I don't think my illness has really compromised my life plans. In fact, I've gone way beyond whatever my goals and dreams were as a kid. I've achieved more than I ever expected in my work life and in my personal life. Maybe cancer gave me the deadlines I needed. Some of my friends can't understand how or why I deal with cancer as positively as I do. I just find it easier not to let it consume me emotionally. Sometimes it gets to me, though. I mean, I know I may have a short life span. I worry about the fact that I may not be around to take care of my parents later on. I realize that they may outlive me, and that's a heavy thought.

My next big project is to start a winter house down in Mexico. I guess in many ways these houses have a healing effect on me. I'm not really sure why that is; I certainly can't explain the psychology behind it. All I know is that it works.

As long as we live and breathe, life beckons us to make a contribution. We've felt the tip of Damocles' sword, and the experience has left us with somber memories as well as profound insights. So how are you going to play life, now that it has dealt you a new hand?

The cards are cut. It's your call.

5

Strong Bonds and Fragile Emotions: Relationships with Family, Friends, and Significant Others

> My fiancé was an incredible source of strength and support during my diagnosis and battle with breast cancer. He couldn't seem to do enough for me. But once I'd recovered from the operation, he told me he was having second thoughts about our wedding plans. A couple of months later, he packed his bags and moved out of our apartment. That was the last I saw of him.
>
> — Karen, three-year survivor

WHEN KAREN, an attractive forty-four-year-old lawyer, shared her story with members of Cancervive, almost everyone spoke up. Regardless of age or background, most survivors had experienced a similar situation with family members or friends, spouses or colleagues. Several people took the opportunity to share their stories: Harry talked about his difficulty fitting back into family life after his long hospitalization; Rebecca was upset by friends and relatives who continued to regard her as an invalid; Sonya worried about how to tell potential boyfriends that she'd had a bout with Hodgkin's disease.

But their stories reflect only one side of the coin. Several members described the ways cancer had actually strengthened and enhanced their relationships: Jack, for instance, told how his friends had rallied to his side just when he needed them most, and Karen explained how her recovery from breast cancer had prompted a reconciliation with her teenage daughter.

Each of their stories underscored how, long after diagnosis and treatment, cancer continues to transform survivors' personal relationships. Since family, friends, and significant others all play an integral part in how you adapt to life after cancer, it is important to be aware of the emotional pitfalls you could encounter in relationships.

Recovery from Cancer: A Family Affair

As a cancer patient, your role was clearly defined. You were expected to feel sick. It was okay — perhaps even necessary — to unplug from the world and its responsibilities. But once you've achieved remission and completed treatment, your status changes. Suddenly you are no longer a cancer patient. You are expected to shed that role as quickly and as effortlessly as a hospital gown. Now that you've been declared disease-free, your family and friends are eager for a return to the status quo. They anticipate that you'll promptly shift gears, rev up, and plow full steam ahead into a continuation of your former life.

But like most survivors, you've probably found that making such a transition is easier said than done. It may take many months before you are fully up to speed. Yet those closest to you may choose to ignore that important coda to your recovery. While throngs of friends and relatives are feting your victory over cancer, you may be the only one to realize that being in remission does not necessarily mean you are back "in the pink."

Harry, for instance, talks about the turbulent time he had readjusting to his former role of healthy person and bread-winner after a lengthy hospitalization for non-Hodgkin's lymphoma. The forty-eight-year-old stockbroker found his family life dramatically altered by his long illness. Once he was back home and out of danger, his family expected him to pick up where he had left off, to be the same husband and father he'd always been. But for Harry, recovery wasn't that simple.

"We've never been what you'd call an Ozzie and Harriet–type family," he told support group members. "We've had our fair share of problems. But after my recovery from cancer, my family really began to come apart at the seams — just at the time I was feeling most vulnerable." Harry explained how changes at home, as well as within himself, made for a rocky return to normal life.

My lymphoma was aggressive, and because I developed a lot of complications, I spent the better part of two years in the hospital. I'll tell you, it really slammed the brakes on my life. Even though we had decent insurance, the long hospitalization wiped out our savings. I couldn't help feeling upset and guilty over that.

What was worse, though, was that I really didn't know how to function as a husband or father anymore. I was no longer the head of the household, the provider. It was tough on all of us, and it changed everything at home. My wife had gone back to her old job in real estate and my eldest daughter, Kimmy, took a year off college and moved back home to help out. Even though my two sons tried not to show it, I could tell they resented having to shoulder more responsibility.

My illness was especially tough on my wife, Jill. We'd always had a pretty good marriage. We both share the same sense of humor, and it's helped us take other family crises in stride. But cancer isn't very funny, and the long siege really wore Jill down. Throughout my illness, she prepared herself for the worst. She put on a good face for the kids, but I suspect they also thought their old man wasn't going to make it.

But I surprised them all, including myself; I pulled through. The first couple of months I was home, I took it real easy and tried to gain back my weight and energy. My boss told me to take as long as I needed to recuperate. That suited me fine; even though I was eager to get back in action, I still wasn't up to it yet. What really surprised me, though, was that my wife and kids weren't terribly sympathetic. Kimmy was having lots of fights with her mother; she didn't like living at home after being away at college for two years. And my sons, whom I'd always been close to, were treating me like a stranger. I remember one day when I asked my youngest, Bruce, to run an errand for me. He just exploded, and said that he was sick of my being sick, that it was time I took care of myself.

Jill and I were having problems too. She was becoming more and more involved at work. She said it was because we needed the money, but I think it was her way of distancing herself from me. We grew apart, and I'm not even sure how it happened. I think part of it was that she was fed up with having to worry about me. Then again, Jill had spent all this time trying to figure out how she would live without me. She was all set to lead her own life, and then suddenly I reentered the picture. I had to try to fit back into a relationship that had gone through all these changes, and it left us both feeling unbalanced.

I know now that part of the problem was me. I had become completely disconnected from my old life. I was accustomed to being a sick person; in a way it spoils you. In the hospital I got used to people doing things for me — all I had to do was push a button. After a while you start thinking that it will always be that way.

But Jill wasn't buying into that mentality. Once I got home, she had to keep booting me in the rear to get me going again. I had a hard time adjusting, and to some extent still am. I felt burdened by my family's needs while I was trying to deal with the prospect of my own mortality. All the old responsibilities, like my job, seemed like such a waste of precious time now. But nobody wanted to hear it, and I think my new attitude left them feeling insecure and angry.

As Harry's story so clearly illustrates, a life-changing crisis like a battle with cancer has a profound effect on every member of the family. When one member is stricken, every other member feels the pain, knows the fear, and suffers the anguish. Many families react by closing ranks and reaching out to one another. For families like Harry's, however, cancer creates seemingly unbridgeable rifts and magnifies misunderstandings, ultimately contributing to a cold war atmosphere at home.

It is comforting to imagine that once your disease has vanished, so too will any family conflicts that erupted in the course of it. But life is rarely as tidy as that. However, families that can remain sensitive and flexible to the special stresses and strains of the recovery period may be able to minimize misunderstandings at home.

READJUSTING TO FAMILY ROLES AND RESPONSIBILITIES AFTER CANCER

Harry discovered that his immediate concern as a survivor centered around the role changes his cancer had imposed on the family. During his long illness his wife, Jill, was forced to take over the role of breadwinner in addition to her roles as wife and mother. His children's lives were also disrupted, and they resented the strains Harry's problems placed on their own fledgling sense of independence. Family tension ran high, and angry outbursts became common.

The domestic stress level escalated when Harry had trouble readapting to the life he had known before cancer. His illness had forced him to relinquish so much responsibility and control that he wasn't sure how to go about fitting back in. But more important, cancer had transformed Harry's outlook on life. Rumblings of restlessness and discontent were affecting his reorientation to the workaday world.

Harry's dilemma is certainly understandable. Postconvalescence letdown is a common experience among survivors. After all, there are few experiences as bracing as a brush with death.

In its aftermath you may almost miss the drama and excitement that accompanied the fight for your life. In contrast, the world of nine-to-five can suddenly seem dull, prosaic.

Like Harry, perhaps you're feeling vaguely dissatisfied with your job, your lifestyle, possibly even your family and friends. To make matters worse, the people around you may not understand your new outlook on life. It might even make them nervous.

Judi L. Johnson is nursing director of the Cancer Center at North Memorial Medical Center in Minneapolis, and co-author of *I Can Cope: Staying Healthy with Cancer*. Dr. Johnson notes that for many people, cancer becomes the harbinger of personal change and growth.

It reprioritizes their values, reshuffles their view of who they are and how they relate to the world. For some survivors, this can lead to dissatisfaction and frustration, a feeling of urgency. For others, that personal transformation results in a new sense of empowerment. It provides them with the opportunity to make the kind of life changes they may have never dared consider before.

But making these changes can be disruptive to those around you — and there's the rub. Christine Perkins, Cancervive's director of social services, says that change is an inevitable — and sometimes essential — part of life after cancer. Getting back into gear can, however, send you off in a direction neither you nor your family were expecting. Perhaps cancer has convinced you that you need to change careers or cities, find a new group of friends, or call it quits with your spouse. These things happen — sometimes all at once — and they inevitably set off an emotional chain reaction at home. What can you do when your need for change conflicts with the wishes or desires of other family members? Perkins says that communication is the key to breaking most domestic deadlocks.

As soon as serious conflicts begin to surface in the family, everyone should sit down and start talking about it. This doesn't mean engaging in a lot of blaming and counterblaming — that's unproductive. Instead, each person might begin by acknowledging how cancer has changed their life. It's important for them to discuss how they are feeling about those changes and what they are willing to do about it. Survivors who, like Harry, have experienced a change in their traditional role are going to feel diminished and perhaps resentful that another family member has taken charge of their former responsibilities. Harry's wife, on the other hand, may feel so overwhelmed that she becomes emotionally unavailable. Their children should also express how they are feeling about having their lives disrupted. All of these issues need to be placed on the table and hashed out in a calm, straightforward manner.

Perkins suggests that during family discussions each member should follow these guidelines:

- *Talk about your feelings using only "I" statements.* Don't generalize how you feel. Try to say "I've been feeling neglected" rather than "You've been neglecting me." The second statement is confrontational and will put the other person on the defensive, and before anyone knows what happened the discussion will have escalated into a full-blown argument. If, however, you simply state that you feel neglected, you are giving the other person enough emotional space to empathize with you and possibly respond by saying, "I'm sorry, I wasn't aware of that. Can we talk about it?"
- *Formulate your thoughts by writing them down.* Before you attempt to discuss matters with your family, find some quiet time to pour out your emotions on paper. Sometimes when emotions are running close to the surface in conversation, it's difficult to keep your thoughts focused and orderly. This can lead to angry accusations that will further damage relationships. The process of writing down your thoughts will help clarify what you want to say and how you want to say it.

It will also give you a chance to take the "buzz" off any anger or resentment you are feeling. If your family is especially volatile when it comes to discussing domestic matters, you may even wish to communicate with one another in written rather than verbal form.

Family discussions should focus on finding solutions, not faults. Members need to determine how they can all work together to accept the changes brought about by cancer and the best way those changes can be integrated into everyday life. But if your troubles continue, by no means should you feel reluctant to go outside of the family for help.

THE LAZARUS SYNDROME

It is ironic that for some families, a patient's recovery from cancer can be as disruptive to their lives as the initial diagnosis.

Although news of your remission will set off an avalanche of joy and relief, it could also unexpectedly trigger another round of stress. For months, possibly years, your family lived in a state of siege, serving loyally as the support squadron in the battle against cancer. Once you are past the acute stage of your illness, they may feel it's safe to let down their defenses, and all the frustration and fear they were suppressing will surface. Family members may react to you with impatience, even resentment, leaving everyone to struggle with feelings of guilt, anger, and remorse.

Then again, some families react in the opposite manner, treating the survivor like some kind of local hero, a secular saint who deserves special treatment. You may find family members going out of their way to overprotect and overindulge you, "stuffing" your needs at a time when you're trying to reestablish a sense of autonomy and independence.

A more familiar scenario, however, is when family members or friends stubbornly refuse to see the survivor as a well person. This reaction is widespread among people who cling to the old myth that a diagnosis of cancer is an automatic death sentence. During your illness family members may have prepared themselves emotionally for what they viewed as the inevitable by engaging in what therapists call "anticipatory grief." Now that you are back among the living — like Lazarus raised from the dead — they aren't quite sure how to treat you. Gradually, as you regain weight and recover your stamina, your family will learn to let go of this view they have of you as an invalid. It could, however, take longer than you'd like. Rebecca, fifty-five, describes how two years after her treatment for melanoma her family and friends continue to treat her as if she was just diagnosed.

Any time a friend or relative calls me they preface the conversation with, "So how are you *feeling?*" I always answer back, "My cancer was two years ago, and I feel just fine, thank you very much." I mean, I might be suffering from indigestion or an ingrown toenail, but other than that I'm doing just great. What they really seem to be asking is, "Do you have cancer again?" Sometimes I get the urge to shove them against the wall and say, "Just quit asking. I'll *tell* you if I'm not feeling fine." No matter what I seem to say, there's always that other perception of me unspooling in their minds. I feel tremendous pressure to be chipper around them, because the minute I appear upset or down about something, they think the worst. It's that underlying attitude that prevents me from feeling like a regular Joe.

This kind of message from family and friends can make letting go of the cancer experience a very difficult task. Then again, when you have the distinct feeling that everyone is second-guessing your chances of survival, you start doubting it yourself. What do you do when family and friends insist on viewing you as an invalid? Dr. Johnson suggests that you try to see the situation from their perspective. Try to understand what it is they are feeling and why. That doesn't mean you have to accept their perception of you. But by understanding it you may be better able to deal with it.

It is your responsibility to tell those who are sending a negative message what effect it's having on you. Say something to your family like, "You're not helping me make the adjustment to wellness by telling me I have to take it easy, or by pampering me, or being overly cautious." Let them know that they can be a boon rather than a burden to your recovery by helping you make plans for the future. This gives everyone a common goal, something to focus on other than cancer, and it allows the family to move ahead of the experience.

That doesn't mean you and your family should fake your feelings and act like perpetual Pollyannas. Life takes on a surreal quality when everyone adopts an attitude of denial. The secret is to open up and talk candidly about each person's emotions — the good, the bad, and the ugly. Still, for many families, that's far from easy.

THE CHEERLEADER APPROACH TO RECOVERY

Survivors like Rebecca and Harry are often hesitant to share their innermost concerns with their families, worried that they will cause unnecessary alarm. As Harry observed, "If I'm acting moody, they immediately think I know something that they don't." With their families and friends watching from the sidelines, Harry and Rebecca feel obliged to take on the role of family cheerleaders.

The urge to protect loved ones from undue anxiety is understandable. But if you are reluctant to discuss any doubts or fears you have, you're probably protecting their feelings at the expense of your own, and sooner or later that's going to trip you up. You won't get the kind of genuine support you need if you can't be open and honest with those closest to you.

Try instead to avoid taking responsibility for the way other people choose to feel.

Sometimes the impulse to cheerlead gets switched around. You may have no hesitation about vocalizing your concerns, but your family and friends prefer to put on a happy face; the last thing they want is to hear about cancer again. That kind of talk, they'll tell you, is self-defeating and unproductive. What you need to project is a positive mental attitude.

For Rebecca, family denial was a major problem.

I'm a talker. Talking about things allows me to make sense of them. But when it comes to cancer my family doesn't want to listen. My husband comes from a long line of deniers, so I can't say anything to him about it. My daughter is a little more open to listening, but after a few minutes she'll say, "Oh, Mom, please don't talk about cancer. It's depressing me." The way my family sees it, if you don't talk about something, then it doesn't exist. I know I can't change their minds. Instead, I've learned to go outside my family to get the emotional support I need. I've developed a network of friends who will listen. It took me a while to accept my family's attitude, but I've also learned to recognize the importance of my own needs.

Virtually every family engages in some amount of denial during a crisis; it's one way of establishing a sense of normality. Once the acute stage of your cancer has passed, your family's overriding impulse may be to put the subject behind them as quickly as possible. They may react to you in unanticipated ways, telling you in so many words, "We're worn out, exhausted. It would be nice if you could forget about cancer and stop worrying for a while." This response is natural enough — we all have our limits — but it can leave you feeling confused and demoralized at a time when you need that extra shot of support. Moreover, you have emotions you need to express, things you want your loved ones to hear. This conflict in attitudes is bound to lead to friction sooner or later.

Through counseling families who are attempting to re-adjust to life after cancer, Dr. Johnson has noted that the cheerleading impulse can be a healthy way of adapting — as long as it isn't taken to extremes.

It is important for a family to work through their fears by establishing hope and optimism. However, it's easy for them to go overboard. When I work with families and see that sort of cheerleading going on, I'll immediately try to point out to them what it is they are doing. I will ask them to look at how they operate as a family under crisis. If they handle all their problems with a "Gee, everything's just great!" attitude, then they are going to deal with the survivor the same way.

But that behavior serves only one purpose: to mask reality. I'll explain how important it is to be optimistic and hopeful, as long as they also allow themselves and the survivor to express the entire range of emotions they are feeling, including sadness and anger. Some families actually need to hear that it's okay to have bad days. Allowing the survivor to talk about cancer can be upsetting to the family, but it's also extremely therapeutic.

Some families need to reach a state of crisis before they feel compelled to begin sorting through their emotions and confronting important issues. If you need to talk frankly about cancer and aren't getting the cooperation and support you need at home, find a nearby sounding board. Locate an empathetic friend, an able therapist, or an available support group.

Let's face it: we all enjoy happy endings, and everyone loves a winner. But life after cancer doesn't always conform to such a sunny scenario, regardless of how much you and your loved ones desire it. Cancer emotionally pressurizes the entire family. An essential part of the recovery period involves allowing everyone to decompress at a rate and in a way that is comfortable for each person. When a family gets stuck it is usually because communication is blocked and emotions aren't being shared.

Cancer is a family affair. It represents a challenge to family unity as well as an opportunity to strengthen bonds and increase love, respect, and understanding. It might help to remind your family that in many ways they are just as much survivors of cancer as you are. Learn how you can work together to make life after cancer as rewarding and as fulfilling as possible. Harry summed it up when he said:

What we went through during my illness was about as scary as anything Stephen King could have written. I know some families fall apart because of cancer, and we were close to that point ourselves. For us, talking it out made all the difference. But someone has to make that first move. Since I was at the center of this crisis, I felt it was my responsibility to try and resolve it. I made a point of setting aside time after dinner for us to talk about what each person had gone through as a result of my illness. We had some arguments, sure, but we also got a lot out on the table.

My family made it clear that they wanted a quick return to normalcy. They wanted the old Harry back. The kids were especially eager to put their fears to rest. They asked me a lot of questions like "Will you get cancer again?" and "What will happen if you do?" I told them that I couldn't promise anything, but that the doctors thought I'd knocked it out for good. I explained that I felt a lot like Rip Van Winkle. It was as if the world had somehow passed me by, and I no longer fit in the same way.

I told them I needed time to adjust, to make some needed changes in my life. My old job didn't interest me anymore. I wanted something more personally fulfilling and less stressful. We went around and around with it, but eventually we reached an understanding. They were willing to support the changes I needed to make, but they made it clear they weren't about to pamper me.

My career decision really upset Jill, since she thought it could jeopardize us financially. We spent a lot of time going over the options until we finally reached a compromise. She enjoyed being back in the work force, and since we needed the income, she decided to continue working. I told her I would stay with the brokerage firm for the time being until I could figure out a new career move.

But Jill and I had a lot more to work on than that. It wasn't easy rebuilding our marriage. There were so many difficult emotions to work through. We started seeing a marriage counselor and that has helped get our relationship back on track.

Kimmy has gone back to school and I can tell she's much happier. My two sons still act a little strange though. I think they're having a hard time accepting that their dad isn't the same guy he used to be. But we talk about everything that comes up and I think it helps reassure them.

It's taken a lot of time and work, but I think we've finally kicked this family back into shape. We're now more appreciative of each other and the time we have together.

Cancer's Effect on Intimate Relationships

Karen, the breast cancer survivor introduced at the beginning of this chapter, began attending Cancervive meetings more than a year ago. The overriding reason for her coming was to make sense out of why cancer had disrupted several important relationships. Karen explained how, shortly after recovering from breast cancer surgery, her fiancé suggested they postpone their wedding plans.

I'd known Philip for several years — or at least I thought I knew him. He wanted to get married a few months after we met, but I wasn't in any rush. I'd been married once before, and I was nervous about taking on that kind of commitment again. Also, I have a fifteen-year-old daughter who wasn't entirely crazy about Philip. But a couple of years later, I changed my mind and accepted his proposal. We got engaged in April and started making plans for a fall wedding.

That summer I found out I had breast cancer. At first I wouldn't accept it. I didn't fit the typical breast cancer profile. I was relatively young, with no family history, and I was in great physical shape. Then the reality of it hit me, and I fell apart. Philip was terrific, though. He calmed me down, convinced me that I was going to be okay, and helped me get through my mastectomy. He was a great source of strength and emotional stability, even though I knew it was hard for him to accept what was happening to me.

My daughter, Tricia, on the other hand, had a tough time with my illness. Before my diagnosis, we'd been having our ups and downs, the usual things you go through with a teenager. When she found out I had cancer, she just closed up emotionally. Perhaps she thought I was abandoning her. She also resented the fact that I was so dependent on Philip for emotional support. The hardest part of my illness was living with the wall of silence between us.

Fortunately, the mammogram had detected my cancer in its early stages, so I didn't require further treatment. During my recuperation from surgery, I began to notice changes in Philip. For example, when he would kiss me, he'd kiss my forehead instead of my lips. Or when I'd talk about doing something in the future, like planning a vacation for the two of us, he was very noncommittal. I'd ask him what was wrong, but he'd give me the "Oh, nothing" routine. I knew big trouble was brewing when, after I'd come home from the hospital, I noticed how he left the room whenever I tended to my incision. At first I thought he might be doing it out of respect for my privacy. But I felt that since I was going to be marrying this man, he needed to share this with me. So I asked him if he would look at my incision, that it was important to me. He said okay, took a quick peek, and then practically ran out of the bedroom. He made a big point of telling me that it wasn't me he was reacting to, that he was just squeamish. But I knew it went deeper than that; Philip was clearly uncomfortable with this major change in my body.

At first I couldn't understand what was going on, since he had been so loving and supportive during the "iffy" period of my illness. I imagine he felt guilty about leaving me at a time when he thought I might die. But now that I was out of the woods, he seemed to have second thoughts about being stuck with what he obviously viewed as damaged goods. I no longer fit his picture of the perfect wife. I'm sure he was handling it the only way he knew how — by keeping me at arm's length. He tried making up for it by giving me presents and taking me out to expensive dinners. But whenever it came down to getting close physically, well, let's say we were both badly disappointed. Things quickly went from bad to worse. Three months after my operation, he packed his bags and moved out.

That just demolished me. I knew we were having trouble, but I had convinced myself that we could work it out. When he left, it was like another part of me had been lopped off; my self-esteem bulldozed into the ground. Most of my friends were supportive and helpful, but I needed more than that. I was in so much pain that I could barely function. Through a mastectomy support group I found the name of a good therapist. She works with women like me who have lost a breast *and* a man to cancer. I spent months working on myself, reading books and talking to other breast cancer survivors. That's what kept me going.

To my surprise, my daughter also played a big part in my recovery. Ever since Philip left, she's been a great source of support. Tricia had been living with her father, but when she heard what happened she called and asked if it was okay to move back in with me. That way she could, as she put it, provide me with a twenty-four-hour shoulder to cry on. Since then, we've been inseparable.

Cancer challenges all relationships, even ones you thought were unassailable. No one can predict exactly how a spouse or lover will stand up to the test. For many couples, cancer provides an opportunity for greater intimacy and understanding, and the intensity of the crisis forges a cast-iron alliance. But not all couples are capable of withstanding such a trial by fire. Perhaps, like Karen, you have survived cancer, but your marriage, engagement, or love affair did not. Was it you, was it cancer, or was it your partner?

Cancervive members who have experienced a variation on Karen's theme of separation report that the breakup usually occurs either around the time of diagnosis or at the end of treatment. If the relationship was already on shaky ground, chances are the other person will bolt at the first mention of cancer. The exit may be physical — suitcase in hand and out the door. Or the desertion can take place on an emotional level, leaving survivors feeling as alone as if their partners had physically abandoned them.

Other couples will pull together to beat cancer, but the considerable strain of that battle drives them apart. In this scenario, a spouse or lover will remain with the patient through the trying times of treatment, only to disappear as soon as cancer has done the same. It is at this point that many people feel it is "safe" to bow out of the survivor's life. Karen speculates on why her fiancé chose this latter course.

I'm sure Philip felt a real obligation to see me through the surgery, that to do otherwise wouldn't be "right." If he'd cut out at the
time of my diagnosis, he would have been haunted by guilt. Instead,
he waited until I was back on my feet. I'm sure he thought that it
would be the kinder thing to do. The truth of it is, his rejection was
a blow almost as devastating as the cancer itself. Clearly, his timing
had very little to do with letting me down easy. It was just easier
for him.

A sense of duty and moral conscience may dictate if and
when a partner chooses to leave, but for you the more important issue is determining how you will handle it if it happens.

Often when a couple attempt to understand why their relationship failed, they are all too quick to make cancer the
culprit. But that's a bit too convenient. Certainly cancer has
a part in the breakup of relationships, but most often it plays
a supporting role. Survivors say that it was the state of their
relationship before their diagnosis which determined what
happened after it. Cancer simply gives the final nudge to relationships teetering on the brink.

When Dr. Judi Johnson counsels couples who are having
relationship difficulties during or after a bout with cancer,
she encourages them to talk only about the dynamics of their
relationship — excluding the subject of cancer.

One thing I hate to see is a couple that blame all their problems on
cancer. Of course, the dynamics of that couple — the way the two
interact and deal with situations — do get exaggerated during a
bout with cancer, as they would in any major crisis. But the couple
should understand that their problems are based on attitudes and
behavior patterns that were established long before the disease entered the picture. They may not have noticed it before, because they
had already — either consciously or unconsciously — worked out a
sense of equilibrium around those patterns of behavior. Each person had a role to play and a set of expectations to meet, and nothing
really disturbed it.

When a life-changing crisis comes along, that equilibrium is
thrown out of whack. Unless the couple have a clear picture of what

the dynamics of their relationship were *before* cancer entered the picture, their first impulse will be to hang any and all problems on it. Chances are their relationship would have reached this point of crisis sooner or later anyway. Cancer just speeded up the process.

Of course, there are problems directly created by cancer and its treatment — infertility, impaired sexuality, altered body image, and injured self-esteem — that have a major influence on how you and your significant other relate to one another, now and in your future together. It is essential that the two of you address these issues beginning at the time of diagnosis and continuing throughout treatment and recovery. By sharing both the troubles and triumphs of cancer, you and your partner will have the opportunity to strengthen bonds of affection, trust, and commitment. Remember that although you are the one who has had cancer, you will be sharing its legacy with those you love. The challenge is to allow that legacy to enhance your relationships, not undermine them.

PICKING UP THE PIECES

What happens when, like Karen, you and your significant other reach an impasse in dealing with the emotional debris that cancer has forced to the surface? Is your relationship worth saving, and if so, how will you begin to repair it? If your relationship is beyond repair, what can you do to take care of yourself?

Christine Perkins offers this advice:

• *Talk it out.* The word *crisis* means a turning point, a crucial time, a moment of opportunity. For a crisis like cancer to be the catalyst for a stronger, more loving relationship, the lines of communication need to be open and in working order. Your partner is probably just as apprehensive about the future as you are. But if you let it, that fear will wear away at your ability to communicate openly and honestly. If you've allowed that to happen, speak up! The only way you can evaluate the changes that have taken place in your relationship is by talking about them.

• *Learn to let go.* Not all damaged relationships can be repaired. Your partner may be unwilling or unable to put any more effort into the marriage or love affair. Don't make the mistake of shouldering all the responsibility. It's easy to think that if you try just a little harder you can change your mate's attitude or behavior. But the only person you can possibly change is yourself. Concentrate less on trying to solve the other person's problems and focus instead on rebuilding your own sense of wellness.

• *Grieve your losses.* Before someone like Karen can mourn the loss of her fiancé, she needs to work through the grief she feels over the loss of her breast. The process of grieving enables us to come to terms with any significant loss that is beyond our control to retrieve. The pathbreaking work of the psychiatrist Elisabeth Kübler-Ross has allowed mental health professionals to recognize the five stages of the grief process: denial, anger, bargaining, depression, and acceptance. Not everyone experiences these stages in this specific order, and you may feel the need to dwell in one stage longer than in others. Take all the time you need to work through the emotions connected to your loss. And don't feel you have to do it alone. Find some means of evaluating what has occurred and how it has altered not just your body, but your view of yourself and others. Take whatever steps you need, such as reconstructive surgery or getting involved in a support group, to put your life back together in a way that satisfies you.

When you lose a part of your body, that loss can be extraordinarily difficult to work through. When you lose the love and trust of a loved one on top of that, you may respond by turning that second loss inward and feeling somehow responsible for it. Don't let that happen. Avoid taking on the extra emotional burdens of guilt and anger. You don't need them, and you don't deserve them.

• *Discover ways to meet your needs for intimacy.* All survivors — particularly those like Karen who have undergone treatment that alters their physical appearance — are confronted with formidable challenges to their body images, their self-esteem, and their sexuality. We all need confirmation of our significance and worth, and never more so than after cancer. And yet you and your partner may feel awkward or nervous about resuming sexual relations. Perhaps your libido has been affected by treatment. Accept the fact that it could take a while before your sexual life is back to where it once was. In the meantime, find ways to express your concerns and understand each other's sexual needs. It's difficult, of course, for most people to talk openly and frankly about their sexuality. But is it better to suffer in silence? If the two of you are uncomfortable discussing sex, try instead to write your thoughts down and exchange notes with your partner. Whatever you do, don't bring your problems to bed with you. A sensitive subject like sex should be discussed in a nonthreatening context — away from the bedroom.

You might find that professional counseling helps accelerate the process of sifting through the more complex and formidable issues, such as low self-esteem and fear of intimacy. For some survivors, it's easier to start that process by interacting with people who share your emotions and experience in a support group.

• *Remember that it takes two to tango.* As you attempt to alleviate the strains in your intimate relationship, ask yourself, "Could *I* be contributing to the problem?" You'd be surprised how often couples overlook this question. For instance, you could be placing a great deal of stress on your significant other if you've allowed yourself to make a "career" out of cancer. One Cancervive member illustrated this point when he revealed how he had used his disease as a trump card whenever his wife disagreed with him on an important issue. "I would remind her that I was, after all, living on borrowed time," he says. "Even though I'd been in remission for two years, I still felt that way. But she was fed up with that excuse."

Also, it is possible that, without even being aware of it, you are sending mixed signals to your mate — signals that will only alienate the two of you. A Cancervive member who had undergone a mastectomy felt so ashamed of her body that she would dress in the closet, out of sight of her husband. He, for his part, interpreted her behavior as a sign that she wasn't interested in sex anymore, and so he stopped making overtures — which, in turn, confirmed her worst suspicion that her husband no longer found her desirable. Since the two of them were uneasy about addressing the issue, this game of second-guessing went around and around until one day they found themselves talking about divorce over morning coffee.

It's dangerous in any relationship to second-guess what the other person is thinking. Don't make assumptions; ask! And be sensitive to how your own actions and attitude may be affecting the relationship.

• *Give it time.* The process of healing a relationship doesn't happen overnight. You and your mate may have different styles of coping, and the rates at which you adjust to life after cancer will undoubtedly be different. Respect those differences and try to stay flexible to each other's needs. Give yourselves time to heal.

Cancer's Effect on Friendships

When cancer slams into your life, your friends are among the first to feel the shock waves. Like buildings shuddering in an earthquake, friendships will undergo a rough-and-tumble test of their strength and durability. Some relationships will come through the trauma no worse for wear; some may even be reinforced, whereas others will have collapsed.

But now that you've beaten cancer, your friends will be recalibrating their perceptions of you. At first they may not know how to react. A few may be so apprehensive about saying the wrong thing that they find it easier to stay away. You in turn will be sifting through your own perceptions of who your real friends are. One of the more difficult decisions you face as a survivor is determining whether or not to salvage damaged friendships. Should you try to repair them? If so, what is the best way to go about it? And if you're single and dating, what part does cancer play in courtship?

These are some of the questions Sonya brought to a recent Cancervive meeting. The vivacious twenty-four-year-old college student says she was unsure of how to deal with the friends she had lost during her battle with Hodgkin's disease two years before. Sonya also worries about revealing her medical history to potential boyfriends.

When I was first diagnosed, I had some pretty disappointing experiences with friends. I was hurt most by my boyfriend, who proceeded to dump me shortly after I was diagnosed. He was completely freaked out by my cancer; he couldn't even say the word. The same thing happened with a couple of my girlfriends. After they heard about my illness, they stopped calling me. Initially, I tried making excuses for them, telling myself that they were just busy. But underneath I knew what was happening.

People my age have a lot of misconceptions about what cancer is really about. There is still a lot of that "get cancer and you die" mentality, and so they act as if I'm this doomed person. I remember telling one date about my illness. I explained how I'd had Hodgkin's disease, and at first he seemed very curious about it. When I told him it was a form of cancer he got totally weird and immediately wanted to know if it was contagious. Needless to say, that was the last I saw of him. Sometimes I wonder under what rock some of these people have been hiding.

There are times when I feel cut off from the social life I used to know. The tough part is deciding how to deal with it out there in the real world. It doesn't bother me that I've had cancer, but it seems to bother a lot of other people. I worry about whether I should put myself on the line, whether it's worth risking rejection. And yet I feel I should tell people about it because, for me, it's important not to base friendships on deceit.

Unlike family members, your friends have no obligation to see you through the hardships of treatment. Their involvement in your life is strictly voluntary. A crisis like cancer is therefore a litmus test of friendship, separating true-blue friends from the fair-weather variety.

Cancervive members frequently talk about how, years after diagnosis, their cancer history continues to set them apart socially. Sometimes this sense of isolation is due to rejection by cancerphobic people, but it can also be self-imposed. Cancer has changed who you are and how you view others, and you may no longer relate to old friends in the same way. A weeding-out process takes place as you decide which friendships still hold meaning for you. As Dr. Judi Johnson explains, sometimes this winnowing is necessary to ensure your well-being.

Many times survivors will shed old friends and gravitate toward people who are going to help, not hinder, their recovery and long-term survival. Your friends can do that simply by being there for you and listening when you need to talk about cancer. Then again, maybe you don't want to talk about it; good friends will respect that too. I would suggest that if you don't have these kinds of friends among your immediate group, then you should either change your social circle or seek out a support group. Find people who are going to contribute to your sense of wellness.

You can find the positive social reinforcement you need at support groups or with one or two faithful friends. But what can you do about the people who let you down or abandoned you?

First of all, try to understand what caused your friend to behave in such an unfriendly way. As you've probably guessed, it's all about fear. People who harbor irrational fears of cancer are likely to shun you if only because they are unsure of how to act or what to say. Your illness may also be an unwelcome reminder of their own mortality. For these people, it's easier to avoid you than to confront such fundamental fears.

RENEGOTIATING FRIENDSHIPS

It's hard to reconcile yourself with people who have ended their friendship with you. Feelings of pride or anger may impede any thoughts you have of reconciliation. And yet, underneath these painful emotions you may feel a strong tug of regret, and with it, the need or desire to reestablish contact. Should you decide to salvage a damaged friendship, Christine Perkins offers the following advice:

• *Try not to hold a grudge.* Friendship requires give and take; if your friend has given you a hard time during your illness, try not to take it to heart. When cancer is involved, you can be sure that the person is reacting to the disease, not to you.
• *Reevaluate the relationship.* Is the friendship worth preserving? If so, why? Do you still have common interests? For instance, a few of your companions may be avid party goers. But if partying is no longer a high priority for you, then you and your friends may choose to go your separate ways. Take the time to weigh the strengths and weaknesses of the relationships you want to reestablish. Ask yourself what it is that you are looking for in a friend. Be as realistic and honest as you can, and let that answer be your guide.

- *Take the initiative.* If you've decided the friendship is worth maintaining, be prepared to make the first move. Your friend may need to know where you stand before approaching you. So make a phone call or drop a letter in the mail. However you make your overture, try not to let anger interfere with it.

- *Begin a dialogue.* Your first impulse may be to ask your friend what happened. Don't be surprised if an answer isn't immediately forthcoming. Most people have a hard time expressing their deepest emotions, particularly when it concerns an issue as fear-laden as cancer. First allow your friends to come to terms with their feelings, then give them the time and space to express themselves.

  Talk about what has changed in your relationship and what you think needs to change. Urge your friends to ask questions about your experience with cancer. This not only breaks the ice but also gives you a chance to clear up any misconceptions they may have. You might find your companions are reluctant to raise the subject, fearing it will stir up unpleasant memories for you. Be open with them about how much you want to share.

- *Know when to let go.* If your attempts at renewing or repairing a friendship don't work out, if your friend doesn't respond to your overtures, learn to let go of that friend. Find a way to work through the emotions of the loss, and then replace that relationship with one better suited to your needs.

Cancer and Dating

Single survivors like Sonya often find that romantic relationships are derailed as soon as their medical history is introduced. Such a rejection can be traumatic to even the most confident survivor. With it comes a profound sense of abandonment and vulnerability, and a disturbing feeling that cancer is shadowing your romantic destiny.

Some survivors prefer to avoid the risk of rejection altogether and will choose to date only other survivors. Then there are those who feel that a cancer history makes no difference in their social lives. They refuse to be anything but up front and honest. These survivors aren't overly concerned about risking rejection; if they can accept cancer, they fully expect their friends to do the same. For them, the issue isn't if they should tell, but rather when to do it.

WHEN TO TELL: IS THERE A RIGHT TIME?

Some Cancervive members think it is essential to reveal their medical history at the first available opportunity. As one man said, "I can't feel completely comfortable with a woman until I know whether or not she's cancerphobic. So on the first or second date I'll tell her pointblank. If she accepts it, then I can relax and feel hopeful that maybe this relationship will work out."

There is certainly nothing wrong with being forthright; it allows you to set the stage for an honest and sincere relationship. If this approach results in high attrition in your romantic life, however, you might rethink your tactics. It could be that you are using this "first strike" approach as a way of protecting yourself. Or perhaps you are using your history of cancer as a way of testing the other person. "I've had cancer; take me or leave me" is the message implicit in this approach. Try to determine what is motivating your need to tell potential partners of your illness. Christine Perkins asks:

Are you trying to protect yourself from making a risky emotional investment, or are you unconsciously looking for ways to reinforce a negative self-image? Then again, it may be that you have allowed cancer to become such an overwhelming part of who you are that you're unable to share yourself in any other way. If so, you might want to ask yourself if that kind of approach is really being fair to you or your friend.

On the other side of this issue are the survivors who have found that honesty is not the best policy — at least not on the first or second date. Experience has shown them that most people are threatened when confronted with the topic of cancer early on in a relationship. It could be that you are hitting your friend with too much too soon — before both of you have had a chance to establish bonds of affection and trust.

There is another advantage to waiting. If, somewhere down the road, the two of you part ways, you will have a better idea as to whether it was cancer or simply "bad chemistry" that caused the romance to sputter out. For many survivors, it is important to make this distinction. But that's hard to do if you have made a point of revealing your cancer early in the game.

The issue of disclosure is a personal one; only you can know if and when to share this part of who you are. Most survivors say it all comes down to sizing up the other person and then gauging whether the relationship has potential for longevity.

HANDLING REJECTION

Suppose you do wait until you've established a sense of rapport and intimacy with your partner. You mention your cancer, and voilà, your date performs a vanishing act. If that person means anything to you, chances are you're going to want to find out why. Perhaps your partner is cancerphobic; if so, you may have little success in renegotiating the relationship. But rejection can be motivated by other, less obvious reasons, and it may help you deal with this painful experience by knowing what they are. For example, some people actually believe that cancer is contagious, or that because of treatment you may now be carrying "bad" genes that could affect your offspring. Or your partner may conclude (in most cases, incorrectly) that treatment has caused you to be infertile. Fear of recurrence is another obstacle that can impede a relationship. Your partner may suspect that because you've had cancer you are destined to die an early death. (Of course, fear of recurrence can work both ways: if you don't have much faith in your future, you'll have a hard time committing to and maintaining a long-term relationship.)

Should any of these issues prevent you and your partner from going forward with the relationship, it's worth the effort to straighten out the misunderstanding. Help your friend see that most cancer-related fears are based on ancient myths and misconceptions. You may even suggest that your partner talk to a physician if you think that would help.

And if your friend still can't handle it? Then it is probably time to say goodbye. It's also time to count your blessings. Says Dr. Johnson:

Aren't you lucky you saw the handwriting on the wall now rather than later? If they can't handle cancer in your past, how would they ever possibly manage if it recurred? How are they going to deal with *any* crisis? It's hardly likely such a person could be there for you. So in a sense, they are doing you a favor by showing you their true colors before you've made a serious commitment.

As painful as rejection is, try not to take it as a personal affront. After all, who did the rejecting? And what was it your friend was reacting to? How did your friend feel toward you before learning about your illness? Answering these questions will help you see that the problem lies not with you, but in your partner's attitude. Also, make no mistake: a clean medical record is no guarantee of a successful romantic relationship. Heartbreak happens all the time to perfectly healthy people. Learn to believe in who you are and what you have to offer others.

Here's what Sonya had to say about it:

I used to think that if guys couldn't accept my cancer, that was their problem, not mine. I felt real militant about it, like I had to blow everyone out of the water just to see who would stick around. But I've mellowed. Now I only tell people when I think they need to know. I've developed a sort of second sense about who can accept that kind of information and who can't or won't.

It's been a couple of years since my cancer, and I've started talking — in very small doses — to some of my old friends about what happened to me. I can be a little more open about it now, mostly because so much time has passed and they aren't as threatened by it. A few still act weird, but I don't fret over them anymore. In my opinion, it's a waste of time and energy. I've come to realize that even if they knew the facts, it still wouldn't change their attitude. They have proven to me that their definition of friendship is 180 degrees different from mine, and so I just let it go at that.

The ironic part is that while cancer has caused some people to be less accepting of me, it's made me much more accepting of others. I feel more mature now, and wiser. Petty things that used to upset me just roll off my back. And cancer has completely refocused my goals and ambitions. I plan to get a master's degree in social work so that I can work with cancer and AIDS patients. Being on the other side of the fence gives you a real understanding of what life's about.

I don't date as much as I used to, mostly because guys my age seem so immature to me now. I've tried meeting people through the Sierra Club and another local environment group. I look for organizations where I think people will have a more accepting attitude about life.

I realize that the people I'm going to have as friends may not be like everyone else. Instead, they are going to be special in the sense that they can understand what I've gone through and are open-minded enough to appreciate it.

A few months ago I started going out with a new guy. At first I didn't tell him about my illness because I thought it was important that we get to know each other first. Then one night, we were having dinner together and he started telling me about his family, and how he had a younger sister with Down's syndrome. He was very sensitive to his sister's needs, so I thought it might be a good time to bring up my cancer. He acted really cool about it and told me how I was so brave to go through something like that. We talked for a long time about all the strange ideas people have regarding those with disabilities and diseases. By the end of that date, I knew this was going to be the beginning of a beautiful friendship.

People Who Need People

When all is said and done, relationships are what matter most in life. Through them we find love and companionship, learn about the world, and ultimately gain a deeper understanding of ourselves. The survivors who shared their stories in this chapter weathered tough times in their relationships with friends and loved ones, and each carried away a special lesson from the experience.

But not all relationships suffer as a consequence of cancer; some of them thrive.

Jack has that kind of story to tell. Now in his fifth year of remission from chronic myelogenous leukemia, the thirty-eight-year-old entrepreneur has a distinctive way of celebrating survival. Each summer, on the anniversary of his successful bone marrow transplant, he plays a round of golf with his friends. But this isn't just any golf game — and this isn't just any group of friends. Jack proudly reports that last year his annual Platelet Open golf tournament raised thousands of dollars for the American Leukemia Society. He explains how, with a little help from family and friends, his fund-raising idea came about.

I was thirty-one when I was diagnosed with leukemia. I had a wife and two kids, with a third baby on the way. When my doctor called me with the news, I sat down and cried my eyes out for about five minutes. And then, just as quickly, I snapped out of it. I immediately made up my mind that I was going to beat this thing. And even if I couldn't, and I only lived the two years the doctors were giving me, I was determined to make them the happiest years of my life. For me, maintaining a positive attitude was the key to getting through cancer. There are victims and there are survivors. The day I was diagnosed, I made up my mind I was going to be in the latter category.

A few months after my diagnosis, my leukemia went into an acute phase. My doctors were able to control it, but they told me that without a bone marrow transplant I probably wouldn't make it. I underwent an autologous, or "self" bone marrow transplant, and it really knocked me for a loop. While I was recovering in the hospital, I learned that a group of my friends and business associates had been donating blood on a regular basis to give me the platelet transfusions I needed to keep my blood clotting normally. I run a family construction business, and while I was out sick my secretary organized a blood donor program for me. All my donor friends wore beepers so that when my doctors knew I needed a transfusion of platelets, the hospital would call my secretary. She would check her donor list and then beep one of the platelet volunteers. A lot of these people lived way out in the suburbs, which meant they had to take time off from work and make the long drive to the hospital to donate blood. The efforts of my friends and family went far beyond what I could ever have imagined. It was an incredible show of love, support, and friendship. Without them I probably wouldn't be here today.

As I was about to turn thirty-five, I decided to throw a party to celebrate both my birthday and my survival. I also wanted to officially thank all my donor friends. I knew that most of my friends enjoyed golf, so I invited the group to join me for lunch and a game at the local country club. After the golf game, I gave each person a red sweater embroidered with the words "Platelet Open." The afternoon was a big success. In fact, everyone had such a good time that they kept asking me, "Where do you plan on taking us next year, Jack?"

That got me thinking. I had survived cancer, and I had a strong desire to show my gratitude, to give something back. Then the idea hit me: why not sponsor a golf game every year and turn it into a fund-raiser? I approached the American Leukemia Society, and that's how the Platelet Open was born. We just held our fourth annual tournament and I'm proud to report that we raised more than forty thousand dollars.

I can't say that having leukemia was a wonderful experience, but for me it resulted in a lot of wonderful things. Cancer clarified what was really important in my life, and I now know how lucky I am to have such a wonderful family and friends. Thanks to them, I plan on having a great life.

6

The Insurance Obstacle

FOR THE ANCIENT GREEKS, life was ruled by fate. They believed that each man's destiny was determined by powers beyond his control, that the course of events was already written.

Most people don't put much stock in that notion today. And yet when it comes to health insurance, cancer survivors feel as if their fate were indeed written — not in the heavens, but in the computer files of insurance companies across the nation.

As a survivor, you undoubtedly feel proud of your victory over cancer. The battle you waged was nothing short of heroic. But that's not how the insurance industry sees it. In its book, a history of cancer makes you a liability, not a hero. You may want to put cancer behind you and get on with life, but that's not always easy. Your insurance problem is there to remind you of it.

You are reminded every time you apply for a health, life,

or disability insurance policy. Before you can say the words "preexisting condition," the verdict that comes sailing back is usually COVERAGE DENIED. You are reminded when premiums on an existing policy skyrocket to the point where you can no longer afford health insurance. If you are lucky enough to secure coverage through your employer, your insurance company may require a long waiting period before it will cover cancer-related expenses. Or the policy may come with an "impairment exclusion" rider, meaning that the insurance company will cover everything except, of course, cancer.

Years pass, and you may come to regard your bout with cancer as your little secret. But don't fool yourself: the insurance industry is in on it. Every medical detail on any insurance application you have submitted in the last seven years winds up in the data banks of that Big Brother of the insurance industry, the Medical Information Bureau (MIB). Located in Boston, the MIB functions much like a national credit reporting bureau. Its vast computer system collects, stores, and shares pertinent bits of medical and nonmedical information (occupation, hobbies, habits) with its 750 member commercial insurance carriers (excluding Blue Cross/ Blue Shield). Member insurance companies tap into the MIB whenever they want to verify the medical history of a new applicant. Information gleaned from the MIB can make or break your chances of obtaining coverage. Call it data bank destiny: when it comes to health insurance, you are the sum of your charts.

The Bottom Line

What can you do? As a survivor you are caught in a double bind. If on the one hand you attempt to conceal your cancer diagnosis on an application form and are later found out, your policy will be canceled and your claims denied. You may even have trouble ever getting insurance again. On the other hand, if you tell the truth, chances are you will be refused coverage — or offered it at extremely high rates.

In short, it doesn't matter how healthy you feel or how positive your doctor's prognosis may be. Once your insurance application is stamped HIGH RISK, your ability to buy protection against the cost of future illness is seriously diminished. As a result, the threat of financial disaster looms just out of sight for many survivors. In fact, a recent study confirmed that the degree of financial strain on cancer patients is directly related to the availability of adequate insurance coverage.

Of course, insurance discrimination is not limited to cancer survivors. People with AIDS, diabetes, multiple sclerosis, and any number of other serious or chronic illnesses are also forced to contend with similar barriers to obtaining insurance coverage. And not every cancer survivor is uninsurable. Your eligibility will depend primarily on the kind of cancer you've had as well as the length of time you've been disease-free.

I received my own rude awakening to the world of insurance at age twenty-three, when coverage under my parents' policy expired. With my cancer five years behind me, I didn't think I'd have any problem locating coverage on my own. My parents were as distressed as I was to discover how wrong that perception was. I unwillingly joined the ranks of Americans who have been forced to "go bare" — the industry's expression for those without coverage. A year later I obtained insurance when I landed a job with a large firm. But when I quit work to start Cancervive, I was once again among the uninsured. Fortunately, my luck soon changed when I married and obtained coverage through my husband's employer. Now whenever I'm asked how I found coverage, I joke that I married Steve for his insurance.

If insurance is supposed to protect us, why are so many

people left unprotected? Insurers say the reasons behind their restrictions boil down to pure financial survival. "People forget that in this country insurance is a business, and that business is selling a product," notes Melanie Marsh, manager of consumer affairs for the Health Insurance Association of America. Naturally, the bottom line is important to insurance company stockholders. To ensure profits, management strives to control costs. One of the ways they do this is by restricting the types of people they will insure — specifically, high-risk applicants.

Who makes these decisions? Insurance underwriters do. Using actuarial reports and studies, they determine what medical conditions constitute a bad or "substandard" risk. The health insurance industry only wants you if you are a "preferred" or "standard" risk — that is, someone who is unlikely to file a lot of claims. And since anyone with a chronic condition has a better-than-average chance of incurring frequent and/or costly medical expenses, that makes you, the cancer survivor, uninsurable.

From the insurance industry's viewpoint, this policy is not discriminatory — it's merely prudent business practice. But to those who can't get insurance, that practice goes by other unprintable names.

Of course, many survivors find adequate and affordable insurance through their employers. But not just any employer will cover you. If you're in search of a generous benefits package, the bigger the organization, the better your chances, because large companies are often covered by group policies where individual underwriting may not apply. If, however, you land a job in a small business (a firm with twenty-five or fewer people), you may be out of luck. Insurance underwriters scrutinize the background of each person covered under a small business policy as closely as they would for an individual policy. If they find a group member with a "high-risk" health history, the insurance company may either decline coverage to the entire group or offer it at exorbitant premiums.

Why are large employer group plans more open to accepting people with a history of cancer? It all comes down to numbers: the greater the pool of preferred premium-payers, the less the financial risk for the insurance company.

Job Lock

For survivors who are covered by employee benefits, insurance problems aren't likely to crop up until they leave their jobs. Unless they can find a new job quickly, one where the insurance underwriter doesn't ask questions about new employees, their search for insurance is likely to be an uphill battle. As a result, survivors often stay in jobs that don't suit them, or for which they are overqualified or underpaid, simply because the job provides the security of affordable insurance. The situation is called "job lock," and it's a common problem among survivors.

I know about job lock firsthand. Eight years after my treatment for rhabdomyosarcoma, I was working as a special events director for a large department store in Los Angeles. I'd spent the last few years working my way up the management ladder. The salary was great, and I appreciated the generous benefits package that came with it. Then one day I received the bad news. My supervisor informed me that the store was undergoing reorganization. My position, along with half a dozen others, was to be eliminated.

I worked with the personnel director, but he couldn't seem to locate any openings for me. I was worried, but losing my job didn't scare me as much as the thought of losing my benefits. I still viewed my health insurance as the only real protection I had against a possible recurrence.

I was so desperate to keep my coverage that I accepted another position at a branch store located more than an hour's drive from my home. There were no openings in the store's public relations department, or any other equivalent management position, so I swallowed my pride and took a job as a salesperson. I knew that I would be underemployed, but at least I'd retained my health insurance.

My story is familiar to any survivor whose insurance coverage is linked to an employer. A young man named Lawrence recently told me about how frustrated he was with his job as a typesetter for a graphics design company. The pay was adequate, the benefits were good, but he'd reached a dead end. After a long search, Lawrence located what he considered an ideal job at a small but growing advertising agency. He scheduled an interview with the personnel director. The meeting went well, and Lawrence was asked to fill out an application. When he did not hear from the director, he called. The position, he was told, went to somebody else. The director explained that Lawrence's cancer history would have driven the firm's insurance premiums sky-high.

Survivors report that there are other drawbacks to company-provided coverage. For instance, what if you are a full-time employee and, because of health or personal reasons, you need to cut back on your work schedule? Since part-timers and hourly wage earners are rarely included in a company's health insurance plan, you're stuck: if you trim your work schedule, you may lose your benefits. Or perhaps you've always wanted to start your own business. Inability to obtain affordable private coverage is likely to douse your dreams of entrepreneurship.

Young survivors who have neither a solid work history nor insurance through parents or a spouse are most vulnerable to job lock. Even healthy individuals can fall victim to it if their dependents fall sick. For example, the father of a child with cancer may feel compelled to stick it out in a dead end job for fear of losing coverage he could have difficulty replacing.

Can anything be done to prevent job lock? Unfortunately, very little. Survivors can sometimes avoid the problem by applying for positions with large corporations or multinationals, where there is safety in numbers. Within large corporations, moreover, survivors have greater opportunities to change jobs without risking termination of benefits.

Job lock is just one of the unfortunate results of insurance discrimination. Until we change the way we handle health care financing in this country, there is very little survivors like Lawrence can do to improve their plight.

Forced Out of the Work Place

Prior to her cancer diagnosis, Lilly worked as a free-lance marketing consultant. She was, she says, "one of those people who never get sick." So instead of taking out an individual health insurance policy, Lilly decided to pay her own medical bills out of a special savings account she set aside for that purpose. Over the years she saved and invested wisely, and she felt financially secure. But she certainly wasn't prepared to handle the cost of a catastrophic illness.

It happened shortly after my forty-third birthday. My doctor called me up and told me that the lump we'd been monitoring in my breast was malignant. After the mastectomy, I was told my cancer was aggressive and had spread to thirteen lymph nodes, and that I had a thirty percent chance of living five years. I was numb with fear — for my life, and for my life savings. I had approximately a quarter of a million dollars in medical bills the year I was diagnosed, covering chemotherapy, radiation, and a bone marrow transplant. It wiped me out financially. I had no choice but to turn to Medicaid. Fortunately, it paid for everything I couldn't pay.

But now I'm stuck. If I go back to work, I'll be disqualified from receiving Medicaid. No insurance company will touch me. I heard about a couple of insurance firms that were still writing minimal policies for survivors who have been treatment-free for six months. I contacted both of them and found out that the underwriter had just changed the waiting period to two years. Even if I could find an insurance company to cover me, I'd never be able to afford the premiums. I've applied for lots of jobs, and they've all told me that they'll cover me under the employee benefits for everything except cancer. But what good does that do for someone like me, who's got a pretty good chance of having a recurrence?

It's been fifteen months since my diagnosis. I'm in a very critical period right now, but so far so good. And even though I feel fine and I'm fully capable of working, I'm forced to remain unemployed just so I can keep the minimal insurance coverage I have under Medicaid. It's like the system has shut me out. It's a very demoralizing situation to be in.

Public assistance programs are available to help those who, caught in circumstances beyond their control, need a helping hand from the government. But some people, like Lilly, find them demoralizing. Unfortunately, millions of uninsured individuals continue to fall through the cracks in our health care system. They don't earn enough to cover the high cost of private insurance, and they aren't poor enough to qualify for Medicaid. When a serious illness strikes, people such as Lilly find that their only way out is to quit their jobs, use up their assets, and apply for assistance.

Caught in the Squeeze

In a free enterprise system such as ours, most of us expect to get what we pay for. We may spend years dutifully doling out insurance premiums. But what we think we have coming to us isn't always what we get.

Like many self-employed people, Frank found that when he went shopping for affordable health insurance several years ago, his options were limited. He learned through a friend that he could obtain coverage by joining a professional organization. A successful photojournalist, Frank joined a national organization for professional photographers and purchased an individual health insurance policy through the group.

This type of coverage is known in the insurance industry as an "association group" policy. But association group insurance is not always the same as the group insurance that employees of a large business receive. Association groups vary widely in the way they are structured. Some offer true group protection and advantages, such as higher benefits and lower deductibles. Others carry none of the advantages of standard group policies. Still, for many people they are an affordable way of obtaining insurance.

Frank was satisfied with his coverage and more than a little relieved to have it when he was diagnosed with colon cancer last year. That's when his insurance problems began.

I was covered under an individual policy, even though my insurance company sold it as part of a group. They were able to do this by combining blocks of individual applicants into groups. It wasn't cheap coverage, and the benefits weren't exactly the greatest, but it was the best I could get for what I could afford.

After I was diagnosed, they removed the tumor and then started me on a course of chemotherapy. That's when I noticed an increase in premiums. I called my insurance company, and they told me that premiums had gone up for everyone in my group. I was told that if, after my chemo, I was in "good health" they would switch me to a different group. That way, they said, I could get a break on my premiums. However, if I didn't qualify medically, then I'd have to stay in the group I was in.

A friend of mine tipped me off to what my insurance company was doing. It turns out that about a year after they open a group policy, they do an assessment of it. If anyone in that group is utilizing benefits beyond a certain level, they start to up the premiums on everyone in that group. If you call the insurance company, they say, "If you are in good medical health, we'll take you out of that group and put you in a new, less expensive group."

I contacted another policyholder who was similarly affected. It didn't take me long to see that my insurance company was trying to dump all the high-risk individuals, and this was their way of doing it.

I've still got coverage, but only for as long as I can pay these ballooning premiums. I've had to take a part-time job at night just to make ends meet. My premium is currently [in 1990] running close to five hundred dollars a month, and I expect it to go up any day now. And I can't do a thing about it.

Frank has become a victim of what is known in the insurance business as "adverse selection." By this method, an insurance company weeds out policyholders who have become bad risks. As Frank found out, first they raise premiums on everyone in the group. When policyholders call to object to the rate hike, they are offered the option of joining another group, one that promises either better benefits or lower premiums. Then comes the catch: policyholders must meet stringent conditions in order to join the new group. Since individuals recently diagnosed with a serious illness obviously do not qualify, they have no choice but to remain in the old group and watch their premiums soar until they can no longer afford coverage.

There are no easy solutions for survivors who find themselves squeezed out of coverage by high premiums. As long as a company's actions do not violate any part of your policyholder's contract, there's not much you can do. However, if you believe that the provisions of your policy are being violated or ignored, you should not hesitate to speak to your insurance agent or some other company representative. Failing that, register a complaint with your state insurance department.

Also, should you decide to change your coverage in any

way, ask your insurance representative to amend your current policy. Be wary of signing any new application intended to convert or supplement an old policy for "better" coverage. And be sure to check any new policy for its preexisting condition clauses. Avoid paying full price for partial coverage.

You Say Prosthetic, They Say Cosmetic

For many survivors, prosthetics are often the Catch-22 of post-cancer care. That certainly was the case for Erin, who at thirty-two is a veteran of cancer.

Diagnosed with a brain tumor at age nine, Erin's cancer treatment included a year and a half of chemotherapy and radiation. She's had two recurrences since her initial diagnosis and is now in remission. The aggressive treatment she received over the years has caused many visible long-term side effects, including permanent alopecia, or loss of hair.

Most people wouldn't consider a wig to be a prosthesis. But if you're a female cancer survivor and treatment has resulted in permanent hair loss, that is exactly what your hair piece becomes. Says Erin:

I tried for years to wear inexpensive wigs, but virtually every wig I bought ended up back in the box. Those wigs just aren't made to be comfortable on bald heads. So now I use a human hair piece that requires replacing every few years. My last replacement cost me twenty-three hundred dollars. That's double what it cost seven years ago. What gets me so mad is that my husband's insurance company refuses to cover more than one prosthetic device. It's a one-time-only deal with them. So every time I need to replace my wig, we go deeper into debt.

I know my bald head is only considered a cosmetic problem, but it's really much more than that. When I try talking to my insurance company about it, they act as though I'm griping about petty stuff. But who are they kidding? Appearances *do* matter. And how many women have to deal with permanent baldness?

Nancy knows the anger Erin is feeling. Three years ago, Nancy lost much of her jaw as well as some facial bone to cancer. In order to speak, eat, or drink, Nancy must wear a custom-made prosthesis. Unable to get a job, she applied for Social Security disability. Because no insurance company would take her, Medicare became Nancy's sole health care supplier.

Last year my medical bills totaled more than seven thousand dollars. A prosthodontist [dentistry specialist] created a prosthesis for me that would work with my remaining facial bone structure.

The income I made last year from my home-based typing service was only five thousand dollars, so I was forced to sell off most of the stocks I'd inherited to cover the cost of the prosthesis. And then I waited to see how much Medicare would reimburse me. Out of the total bill, they paid only sixty dollars.

I was sure they'd made a mistake. I immediately contacted my doctor and the local Medicare office. But there was no mistaking that amount. As it turns out, it all comes down to language. The people at the Medicare office told me that my inter-oral prosthesis is considered dental work, and Medicare doesn't cover any kind of dental work. And yet without that so-called dental work I can't use my bionic part, and that means I can't eat or talk properly. If I had lost a breast to cancer, I'd have been reimbursed not only for a new breast prosthesis, but also for the cost of four brassieres a year. It just isn't right to deny the cost of basic functions to one cancer survivor while providing cosmetic prostheses to others.

All I have left in the way of assets now is my house. If I need another inter-oral prosthetic device, I'll have to take out a second mortgage. But what choice do I have?

Some states now require certain types of insurance protection for post-cancer care, such as that mandated in a provision added to the California Insurance Code in 1978. Under this amendment, all group disability policies that provide coverage for mastectomies must also provide for either breast prostheses or breast reconstruction. But those who have had mastectomies are a small percentage of the total population of recovered cancer patients, and there are many other kinds of prosthesis which are just as if not more important to the well-being of survivors.

According to Melanie Marsh, insurance companies vary widely in their reimbursement policies for prosthetics.

Cancer survivors need to keep in mind that each state has its own rules and regulations regarding how insurance companies operate within that state, so what may be true in one state may not apply in another. Also, some companies are more liberal in their reimbursements than others. Most policies refer to reimbursement of items that are considered "medically necessary" or that fall under the heading of "standard medical practice." But the definition of those terms varies from one company to the next.

Reimbursement for prostheses has always been a slippery area with health care insurers. What you may consider necessary and essential to your recovery may not be deemed such by the powers that be. It's easy to see how an insurance company might decline Erin's claim on the grounds that a new hair piece is nothing more than a cosmetic device. But for survivors like Erin, a hair piece is essential to their emotional recovery.

What is even more perplexing is Medicare's refusal to reimburse Nancy for the reconstructive work done on her mouth — even though without her inter-oral device she cannot use the prosthesis that allows her to eat and talk. Says Marsh:

There are a number of insurance plans that, because they don't cover dental, have trouble reimbursing for any kind of mouth work. You actually have to prove to them that it is not dental or cosmetic work, that it is instead medically necessary surgery. I would advise anyone in a similar situation to obtain documentation from their doctor and appeal the decision.

As with most barriers to insurance coverage, there are no clear-cut solutions to the problem of reimbursement for prostheses. You should, however, obtain a copy of your insurance contract and study it. Find out what it will and will not cover. If you have trouble with claims reimbursement or suspect the insurance company is violating your policy in some way, there are a few things you can do.

- *Learn the lingo.* Understand the language insurance companies speak. Before you submit a claim for a hair piece, for instance, ask your doctor to write a "prescription" for it. Make sure the prescription specifically uses the term *hair prosthesis* and not *wig* or *hair piece*. Similarly, when you buy your hair piece, insist that the receipt also state that it is for a hair prosthesis, not a wig. Remember that this documentation will be the basis for your claim for reimbursement.
- *If your claim is denied, resubmit it.* Ask your doctor to write a letter detailing why your claim is justified and include it with your appeal. If your second try fails, submit it yet again. Let the company know that you intend to be tenacious about your insurance rights.
- *Get on the phone.* If your claim continues to be denied, talk to a supervisor in the claims department of your insurance company. Your reimbursement problem could be the result of an administrative mix-up. Sometimes a phone call to the insurance company (or asking your doctor to make the call) is enough to clear up the problem. Follow up any phone calls you make with a letter to the claims supervisor recapping the conversation and restating the problem. Include a copy of your original claim along with copies of any additional material that supports your claim.
- *File a complaint.* If you aren't getting a satisfactory response from your insurance company, consider filing a formal complaint with your state's insurance department. Write the de-

partment a letter describing your problem and include a copy of your claim. It is the job of this watchdog agency to set the standards and enforce the rules and regulations of insurance companies doing business within your state. If the department agrees with your claim it may put pressure on your insurance company. Also, be sure to mail a copy of your letter to your state representative or senator.

• *Appeal the decision.* Many insurance carriers have what is known as an appeals process. If you are still getting the runaround, inform the company that you want to appeal its decision regarding your claim. Should the appeal be decided in favor of the insurance company, you can request an outside "peer review" in which an independent panel of physicians and insurance representatives will investigate your claim, evaluate the case, and render a decision.

• *Take legal action.* If the appeals process fails and your state insurance department sides with your insurance company, you have one option left: take your claim to court. (Depending on the amount of the claim, it might be more advantageous to file in small claims court and thus avoid legal fees.) If you decide to retain a lawyer, find one who specializes in insurance litigation. Your best bet, should you choose to pursue legal action, may be to file suit for either bad faith or breach of contract — but your lawyer will know best. You should also consult your lawyer before taking steps or threatening your insurance company with any kind of action. Of course, taking legal action is neither cheap nor easy. But it is sometimes the only way to make a difference. After all, it's the squeaky wheel that gets the grease.

A word of warning for survivors covered under an employer's group plan: when it comes to taking legal action against an insurance company, recent court decisions have stacked the deck against policyholders. Under a law passed in 1974 known as ERISA (the Employee Retirement and Income Security Act), courts have ruled that plaintiffs filing suit against insurance companies can only attempt to recover the benefits lost. In other words, if the suit is successful, plaintiffs are limited to collecting the amount owed the health care provider (they cannot win damages). Lawyers' fees in such cases are awarded at the judge's discretion — so proceed at your own risk.

Ways Around the Insurance Obstacle

Insurance companies are not known for their flexibility. Once underwriters have decided how they're going to rate you, they have a hard time changing their minds. Even if your cancer is ten or fifteen years in the past, the insurance industry may act as if you were diagnosed yesterday. As a consequence, your chances of obtaining coverage through an individual or small company health plan may be slim — but not necessarily impossible.

Survivors should remember that the insurance industry is regulated on a state-by-state basis. Each state has its own department of insurance, and the rules and regulations that apply in one state are often quite different from those in another state. The policies and practices of insurance companies are just as varied. There are no across-the-board answers when it comes to locating coverage. But there are a few general strategies you might find helpful. Here's how you can best weave your way through the insurance obstacle course.

GET A JOB

One of the more tantalizing aspects of working for a large corporation is the generous benefits that come with the job. For survivors, landing a job in a large company is often the easiest way of gaining access to health insurance since businesses with more than twenty workers are required by law to provide employees with health benefits. Also, most group plans offer comprehensive (covering all illnesses) and catastrophic coverage, a must for survivors. Some businesses have "guaranteed issue" plans in which individual underwriting doesn't apply, and therefore no medical questions are asked of applicants. If the plan does require an evaluation of applicants, it's possible that your preexisting condition will be excluded from coverage for a designated waiting period, anywhere from two months to a year. After that you're free and clear. As mentioned earlier, one of the problems inherent in employer-based benefits is that you may fall prey to job lock. Remember, however, that the bigger the company, the greater the chance of job mobility within the company.

A word of caution: because of the rising cost of insurance, more companies are beginning to "self-insure." That is, instead of relying on an outside indemnity plan, these businesses pay for employee benefits themselves. However, companies that self-insure are not required to follow state insurance regulations. If you work for one of these firms and have a problem with your insurance coverage, you may have a more difficult time getting your problem resolved.

What should you do if you are changing jobs? Before you make your move, check up on the kind of benefits you'll have at your new job and if the group policy requires a waiting period for new employees. Explore your old policy for any conversion options or extensions that will cover you during this waiting period. Also, whenever you interview for a new job, make it a point to inquire about the company's benefit package. You might even ask if it is possible to look at a copy of the master policy, just to see what the fine print has to offer. But be sure to inquire about specifics only *after* you've been offered the position. After all, your employer wants to think that your primary interest is in the job — not the fringe benefits.

IF YOU LOSE YOUR JOB

If you lose or quit your job, will you automatically lose your coverage under the company's group plan? Under the federal Consolidated Omnibus Budget Reconciliation Act (COBRA), passed in 1986, employees who leave a firm can now file for an extension of their group coverage.

Companies with twenty or more employees are required by COBRA to provide continuous coverage (regardless of any preexisting conditions) for up to eighteen months to any employee who either quits, is terminated for reasons other than gross misconduct, or is forced to work reduced hours. Coverage under COBRA also extends (for up to thirty-six months) to the divorced, separated, or surviving spouse of that employee as well as any eligible dependents. Although you will have to pay the full cost of this extended coverage yourself, the premiums cannot exceed 102 percent of whatever the applicable premium is for the previous employer's group plan. Once you obtain new coverage, you must relinquish your old policy under COBRA *unless* your new one is limited or carries a preexisting condition clause excluding your cancer. If so, you may use COBRA for up to eighteen months to cover the waiting period required by such a clause.

Keep in mind that COBRA coverage is not automatic. It is up to your employer to inform you of your COBRA rights no later than fifteen days after your group coverage is terminated. Then the ball's in your court; you have sixty days to apply (in writing) for an extension.

You may be interested in knowing that the passage of COBRA's insurance provisions is due principally to the lobbying efforts of cancer survivor and women's rights activist Tish Sommers. When she and her husband divorced in the early 1970s, Sommers, then fifty-seven, was dropped from the health insurance policy provided by her husband's employer. At that time, group coverage did not extend to divorced or

separated spouses. That's when Sommers, a fifteen-year survivor of breast cancer, began her crusade to secure protection
for women who lose their husbands — and their coverage —
because of death, divorce, or separation.

Survivors who think they have been denied their rights
under COBRA should first try to settle any disputes with
their employers. Failing this, they should write to the Pen-
sion and Welfare Benefits Administration, U.S. Department
of Labor, 200 Constitution Avenue N.W., Washington, D.C.
20210.

LOCATE AN INDEPENDENT BROKER

If you are self-employed, or you can't get insurance coverage
through work, an independent insurance broker may be able
to locate a reasonable insurance package for you. Seek out
an agent who specializes in finding policies for high-risk
individuals. But keep in mind that agents and brokers earn
their commissions from insurance companies, not applicants.
Therefore, caveat emptor: let the buyer beware. Agents most
often have your best interest at heart when they suggest an
insurance plan, but be sure that it's the right plan for you.
Educate yourself by asking questions and getting multiple estimates. If necessary, talk to a lawyer or an independent insurance consultant.

Arthur A. Abelson, a survivor of lymphoma, is a chartered life underwriter and financial consultant with the Los
Angeles–based Associates in Financial Planning Group. He
advises survivors to find an aggressive and knowledgeable
broker who will thoroughly research the market and then ne-
gotiate their applications with underwriters.

The problem survivors face is that they are excluded at the insurance underwriter's desk. Most underwriters look only for ways to

keep a high-risk applicant out rather than for ways to allow that applicant coverage. When it comes to filling out an insurance form, I've seen too many survivors merely check off the box that says they've had cancer without qualifying what type of malignancy it was or how long they have been disease-free.

To be sure, insurance forms leave little room for elaboration about a medical condition. But what if your bout with cervical cancer was seven years ago, and since then you've been treatment-free and in excellent health? That information could change your chances. How do you call attention to it? Abelson suggests that your agent attach a letter to the application indicating your present state of health. Include a note from your physician as well as any medical records that will support your agent's letter. This information will allow the underwriter to have a clearer and more complete understanding of your health status. Abelson is quick to point out that although this approach won't guarantee your success in finding coverage, in some instances it can make a difference.

Tips for Filling Out an Application. Too many consumers meekly accept whatever judgment the insurance company passes on them. But what is an insurance application? It's the basis of a contract between you and the insurance company. And contracts are always negotiable. Abelson suggests that survivors keep in mind these points of negotiation when it comes time to fill out the application:

• *Ask your agent for a list of the company's underwriting rules.* Before you fill out an application, ask yourself this question: Do I know how this insurance company is likely to rate me? You'll know where you stand long before you've filled out the application if you review the underwriting policy. You might think checking on the company this way is sneaky, but it is perfectly within your rights to do so. And after all,

Cancervive

don't you want to present yourself in the best possible light?

- *Don't volunteer unrelated information.* Some survivors view their victory over cancer as a badge of courage, and as a result they end up divulging superfluous details. Try to refrain from doing this; it may confuse the underwriter and jeopardize your chances of getting coverage.
- *Get a checkup.* If your agent thinks it will improve your chances, agree to take a physical examination and submit the results to the insurance company. Use whatever ammunition you have at your disposal. Don't forget that the processing of insurance applications is a high-volume business. Unless you call attention to special circumstances regarding your health, your application is apt to be treated in assembly-line fashion.
- *Don't take no for an answer.* Every insurance company has an appeals process. If you think you weren't given a fair shake, get in touch with your agent and say that you want to appeal the underwriter's decision. Keep in mind that even though one underwriter refused your application, that doesn't mean they all will. Insurance underwriters vary in their requirements, depending on the applicant's status and the insurer's risk capacity. Once your broker finds a company that will take you, be sure the company is financially sound and has a reputable service record. One way to check is in *Best's Insurance Reports — Life/Health,* published annually by the A. M. Best Company and available in most public libraries.
- *Steer clear of "cancer insurance."* Be on the lookout for anyone trying to sell you cancer insurance, also known as "dread disease" insurance. As desirable as this kind of policy sounds to a cancer survivor, it often comes with a very high price tag and has a poor return on claims. Again, as with any policy, closely examine the language and fine print on this type of insurance. You may not like what you find. Hospital coverage is often inadequate and may not include cancer-related

costs, such as any illnesses or side effects caused by treatment. Also, these policies usually come with strict limits on how much the company will pay for cancer treatment. Because of the highly dubious nature of these policies, cancer insurance is now banned in several states.

RISK POOLS

Another insurance alternative includes state-mandated risk pools. Nineteen states now offer comprehensive health insurance programs to people who cannot otherwise obtain insurance because of health history or a preexisting condition. Risk pools are created by state legislation, which requires all insurance companies and health maintenance organizations operating within the state to pool their resources and provide comprehensive coverage to high-risk individuals. One of the participating organizations is then appointed to administer the pool and is responsible for handling all the paperwork, including applications, premiums, and benefits. But not just anyone can join a pool. You can qualify for coverage only if you are a resident of a state that offers risk pool insurance.

Unlike commercial carriers, state risk pools are virtually equal in what they offer policyholders. Most pools provide for lifetime maximum benefits ranging from $500,000 to $1 million as well as a choice of deductibles and an 80/20 co-insurance provision (that is, after the deductible is met the pool pays 80 percent of your medical bills and you pay the remaining 20 percent up to a designated maximum. If your expenses go higher than this maximum, the pool will cover 100 percent). Many pools also require either a six-month or one-year waiting period for preexisting conditions.

The down side to risk pool insurance is the price tag. Depending on the state, risk pool premiums can run 125 to 200 percent higher than what comparable coverage would cost a standard-risk applicant. Although these premiums are by no means cheap, risk pools do offer comprehensive coverage that includes inpatient hospital services and physicians' fees as well as costs for some home health care and prescription drugs.

Risk pools won't solve every survivor's insurance problem. Expensive premiums make this type of coverage prohibitive to many people. But for some, risk pools can make a difference.

State High-Risk Health Insurance Pools. Listed below are the contacts for states currently offering risk pool programs. Several risk pools were not yet operational at press time. Call your insurance representative or state department of insurance for information on start-up dates. If you would like to see a risk pool established in your state, write to your state legislature.

CALIFORNIA*
California Department of Insurance Consumer Hotline
(800) 233-9045

COLORADO*
Colorado Department of Insurance
(303) 866-6425

CONNECTICUT
Health Reinsurance Association of Connecticut
Travelers Insurance Company
(203) 527-5369

FLORIDA
Mutual of Omaha
(800) 422-8559

*Risk pool program not yet operational.

GEORGIA*
Georgia Department of Insurance
(404) 651-6993

ILLINOIS
Illinois Comprehensive Health Insurance Plan
Mutual of Omaha
(800) 456-0224

INDIANA
Indiana Comprehensive Health Insurance Association
Blue Cross/Blue Shield of Indiana
(800) 552-7921
(317) 576-6600

IOWA
Comprehensive Health Insurance Association
Mutual of Omaha
(800) 445-8603

LOUISIANA
Louisiana Department of Insurance
(504) 342-5301

MAINE
Maine High Risk Health Organization
Mutual of Omaha
(800) 456-0224

MINNESOTA
Minnesota Comprehensive Health Association
(612) 456-5290

MONTANA
Montana Comprehensive Health Association
(406) 444-8200

*Risk pool program not yet operational.

NEBRASKA
Nebraska Comprehensive Health Insurance Pool
Blue Cross/Blue Shield of Nebraska
(800) 356-3485
(402) 390-1814

NEW MEXICO
New Mexico Comprehensive Health Insurance Pool
Blue Cross/Blue Shield of New Mexico
(800) 432-0750
(505) 292-2600

NORTH DAKOTA
Comprehensive Health Association of North Dakota
(701) 282-1100

OREGON
Blue Cross/Blue Shield of Oregon
(503) 220-6363
(503) 373-1692

SOUTH CAROLINA
Blue Cross/Blue Shield of South Carolina
(803) 736-0043

TENNESSEE
Comprehensive Health Insurance Pool
Mutual of Omaha
(800) 445-8603
(615) 755-6210

TEXAS *
Texas Board of Insurance
(512) 463-6425

*Risk pool program not yet operational.

UTAH*
Utah Department of Insurance
(801) 538-3800

WASHINGTON
Washington State Health Insurance Pool
Mutual of Omaha
(800) 456-0224

WISCONSIN
Wisconsin Health Insurance Risk and Sharing Plan
Mutual of Omaha
(800) 228-7044

WYOMING
Blue Cross/Blue Shield of Wyoming
(307) 634-1393

BLUE CROSS/BLUE SHIELD ASSOCIATIONS

In several states, Blue Cross/Blue Shield offers annual open enrollment periods, when high-risk applicants are accepted regardless of their medical history. However, many of these plans require a waiting period (from six months to one year) before they will cover you for a preexisting condition. As with risk pool insurance, premiums for the "Blues" plans are high and vary from one plan to another. Periods of open enrollment also vary from state to state. For further information, check with your local Blue Cross/Blue Shield company or call your state insurance department.

States Offering Blue Cross/Blue Shield "Open Enrollment" Periods

DISTRICT OF COLUMBIA
Blue Cross/Blue Shield of the National Capital Area
(202) 484-9100

Year-round for residents of Virginia; July for residents of the District of Columbia.

MARYLAND
Blue Cross/Blue Shield of Maryland
(800) 992-2308
(301) 581-3400
June 1–30; December 1–31.

MASSACHUSETTS
Blue Cross/Blue Shield of Massachusetts
(617) 956-4000
Year-round. Some restrictions apply.

MICHIGAN
Blue Cross/Blue Shield of Michigan
(517) 699-3200
Year-round.

NEW HAMPSHIRE
Blue Cross/Blue Shield of New Hampshire
(603) 228-0161
Year-round.

NEW JERSEY
New Jersey Blue Cross/Blue Shield
(201) 822-4500
Year-round. Twelve-month waiting period for preexisting conditions.

NEW YORK
Empire Blue Cross/Blue Shield
(212) 490-4141
Year-round.

NORTH CAROLINA
Blue Cross/Blue Shield of North Carolina
(919) 489-7431

Year-round. Twelve-month waiting period for preexisting conditions.

PENNSYLVANIA
Blue Cross/Blue Shield of Pennsylvania
(215) 241-2400
Year-round. Twelve-month waiting period for preexisting conditions.

RHODE ISLAND
Blue Cross/Blue Shield of Rhode Island
(401) 831-7300
Enrollment period varies, but is usually offered in the late fall of each year. Seven-month waiting period for preexisting conditions.

VERMONT
Blue Cross/Blue Shield of Vermont
(802) 223-3494
January–March.

VIRGINIA
Blue Cross/Blue Shield of Virginia
(703) 342-7352
Year-round. Twelve-month waiting period for preexisting conditions. Other restrictions apply.

JOIN A GROUP OR ASSOCIATION

So you've never been a joiner? It could make a difference in your search for insurance. Many professional, fraternal, civic, and trade organizations offer group insurance to their members. If you're a college alumnus, why not join your alumni association? If you are age fifty or older, look into the American Association of Retired Persons. Organizations like these frequently offer health plans to their members, some of which don't require medical underwriting.

How do you go about tracking down such an organization? To start, make a trip to the reference section of your library and ask for a book called the *Encyclopedia of Associations*. Look up the organizations that most appeal to you. Then contact them to find out the kind of insurance, if any, they offer members. But be careful. Some of these plans are better than others, and premiums can vary dramatically. While you are shopping around, remember to look for a plan that offers comprehensive coverage.

FIND OUT WHAT THE GOVERNMENT CAN DO FOR YOU

At one time or another, most Americans will qualify for some kind of government assistance. Veterans of the armed forces, for example, are eligible for medical care in Veterans Administration hospitals. Disabled people unable to work for a living can qualify for Social Security disability insurance. Because of the difficulty in securing commercial insurance coverage, many survivors who qualify turn to public entitlement programs such as Medicare or Medicaid for their health care needs.

Medicare. Medicare is a government-sponsored health insurance program for the elderly (persons aged sixty-five and older) as well as those who are permanently disabled and have received Social Security disability benefits for at least two years. All employers and their workers pay into Medicare through payroll taxes.

The federal Rehabilitation Act of 1973 classifies cancer as a disability. As a survivor, you may qualify as a "totally disabled" person and would therefore be eligible for coverage under Medicare. Find out what you are entitled to in the way of government help, and then be persistent about getting it.

Keep in mind that Medicare does not provide comprehensive coverage; it is designed only to assist with the payment of medical bills. You may have to look elsewhere to fill in the gaps in coverage. If you are interested in finding out more about Medicare, contact your local Social Security Administration office, which will provide you with information regarding eligibility and how to apply.

The Medicare program is divided into two parts: hospital insurance (part A) and medical insurance (part B). If you apply for hospital insurance under part A, you will be required to participate in Medicare's medical insurance plan under part B as well, for a monthly fee. If you are eligible for Social Security, benefits under part A are free; if not, you'll be required to pay extra for them. Both plans require patients to cover some medical expenses.

- *Part A — Medicare hospital insurance.* This part of the Medicare program provides limited coverage for approved inpatient hospital care, some medically necessary home health care, skilled nursing facility care, and hospice care. Co-payments (where the insured pays a percentage of costs) and deductibles do apply. As of the beginning of 1991, Medicare will pick up the tab on the first sixty days of hospitalization once you've met the deductible.
- *Part B — Medicare medical insurance.* Part B primarily covers doctors' services as well as several other types of medical expenses not covered under part A such as diagnostic tests, administered drugs, and outpatient hospital care. Medicare covers 80 percent of what it considers approved services and "reasonable" charges. Under part B you must pay an annual deductible as well as a monthly premium. To be covered under part B, you must enroll in the program no more than three months after you become eligible for Medicare. For part A beneficiaries who miss this deadline and still wish to

sign up for part B, Medicare offers an annual open enrollment period from January 1 through March 31.

Medicaid. As a last resort, survivors sometimes turn to Medicaid, the health care program funded jointly by federal and
state governments for low-income persons. Medicaid provides for inpatient hospital care as well as outpatient services,
X rays and other laboratory tests, skilled nursing facility care,
home health care, and the cost of transportation to and from
the recipient's health care facility.

If you are unemployed or can prove that you are medically
needy, it makes sense to find out what kind of state benefits
you are entitled to under Medicaid. Rules covering eligibility
and payments vary from state to state. To find out if you are
eligible, contact your local Social Security office or state office
of human services.

HEALTH MAINTENANCE ORGANIZATIONS

Survivors who are not covered by group health insurance at
work should determine if they can qualify for enrollment on
an individual basis in a local health maintenance organization. HMOs are organizations of health care providers which
offer comprehensive medical services on a fixed, prepaid
basis. Members of an HMO pay regularly into the plan and,
in return, are entitled to the medical services of participating
hospitals and doctors. Many employee benefit programs now
include prepaid health plans like HMOs and PPOs (preferred provider organizations). A few of these plans have no
preexisting condition clauses.

Federally qualified prepaid health plans are prohibited by
law from screening group members, although they are allowed to screen people who apply for individual membership. Once an individual applicant is accepted, the HMO can-

not restrict or deny coverage for a preexisting condition. It may, however, require a co-payment arrangement whereby the member pays for a percentage of the services rendered for a preexisting condition. The law also forbids federally qualified HMOs from canceling a subscriber because of high utilization of services.

One of the advantages of an HMO is that, by maintaining its own medical facilities and staff, it offers subscribers one-stop health care. However, HMO members are required to use only those doctors and medical facilities that are members of the plan. This restriction can be a drawback for survivors who don't want to relinquish long-standing relationships with physicians who are not members of the HMO.

LIFE INSURANCE

Survivors often find that life insurance can be as difficult to secure — and as expensive to buy — as health insurance. Most life insurance companies evaluate recovered cancer patients' applications based on the type, grade, and stage of the cancer and the length of time they've been in remission. If you already had a private life insurance policy in place before you were diagnosed, you cannot be canceled because of your illness (unless, of course, you stop paying your premiums). If your life insurance is part of your employment benefits package, however, you may have difficulty renewing that policy once you leave your job. Should your firm allow you to convert to an individual policy, most life insurance companies require you to initiate the conversion within a short time after leaving the position.

To find out which life insurance companies will consider high-risk applicants, check with your local library to see if it has *Who Writes What in Life and Health Insurance*. This annual guide, published by the National Underwriters Company, lists insurance companies by risk categories, such as medical conditions and occupations.

Before you begin to shop, try to find an independent insurance representative to act as your broker and advocate. (You can locate one through your state insurance department or the American Council of Life Insurance, whose address is listed at the end of this chapter.) An independent broker will simplify your search and save you lots of time and trouble.

Be sure to ask your broker to submit your case on a trial application basis. To run a trial application, you and your broker should compile an accurate and up-to-date profile of your current health status. You may be asked to provide any necessary medical records that will substantiate your case. *Without* including your name, Social Security number, or any other identifying information, the broker will then pitch your case to those insurance companies that are likely to be most receptive to you.

It is extremely important that the broker keep your identity anonymous during the trial application period. Otherwise, if the first company your broker approaches refuses you coverage, you will be automatically rated and entered in the files of the Medical Information Bureau. Once that happens, your chances of getting insurance through another carrier will be severely restricted. Using the trial application approach, your broker can determine who will offer you coverage, and at what price, without jeopardizing your chances. When you do find a company that will insure you, be sure to read the policy carefully. Know what you are getting — or not getting — before you sign on the dotted line.

The Need for National Health Insurance

You don't have to look very hard to see that the American system of health care is in critical condition — and sinking fast.

Currently there are an estimated thirty-seven million Americans who are without health insurance — approximately 15 percent of the population. Add to that the millions more who are underinsured, that is, those with skimpy benefits, or with riders or waivers attached to their policies. One study notes that as many as 50 percent of those who are insured are actually underinsured.

As we head into the twenty-first century, the United States remains the only industrialized country in the world (besides South Africa) without a national health insurance program. Instead we continue to rely primarily on private industry to provide a public need.

As a result, far too many cancer survivors (as well as others with serious medical conditions) find that the current system undermines their chances for leading a healthy and happy life. According to consumer advocate Ralph Nader, the goal is clear: "We need to completely replace our present system with a fair and comprehensive program of health insurance that will cover everyone and will emphasize quality control, cost control, and preventative medicine."

National health insurance is not a new idea. Politicians have been batting it around Congress for decades. Although public opinion polls reflect that most Americans believe the financing of our health care system needs an overhaul, no one seems to know exactly how or when it will happen. Washington may eventually get around to revamping the system, but if past political battles are any indication, legislation is likely to languish until the situation reaches catastrophic proportions.

Observes Ralph Nader:

If people think we can leave the health care problem to a few senators to fix, they're wrong. The best chance we have of changing the system is through consumer advocacy, and by convincing citizens that real power lies in grass roots organizations. People have to begin rallying 'round the proverbial village square. Each town needs to organize its own cooperative health clinics. If universal health in-

surance is going to work at all, it must emerge from local community organizations that extend all the way up to the national level.
That way, by the time a universal health insurance law is passed, the
program will have a solid base at the community level.

Cancer survivors deserve decent health care. Health is too
precious to be held hostage to the whims and ways of a
market-driven system of health insurance. National health insurance isn't going to bring about a utopia in health care, but
it just might give us the chance we need to rearrange our
medical priorities.

TAKING RISKS

Insurance reform can't come fast enough for the vast majority of cancer survivors and their families. But the insurance problem is likely to get worse before it gets better. That
doesn't mean you should throw up your hands in despair and
accept the role of victim. A fatalistic mindset isn't very condu-
cive to change. Of course, it's easy to feel as though you don't
have a chance against the monolithic insurance industry. But
don't forget that all it took was one well-placed stone from
David's slingshot to bring Goliath down.

One of the objectives of this book is to stimulate survivors
to self-advocacy. If we are to take charge of our own lives, we
need to educate ourselves and others to the issues that concern us. We need to speak up and take risks.

Irene Card is president of Medical Insurance Claims, a
claim-processing firm in Kinnelon, New Jersey. Long an advocate of survivorship issues, she maintains:

We have to find ways of educating the insurance industry when it
comes to cancer. They still view it as the "Big C." To them, all cancer
survivors are alike: they only live a few years past treatment and
during that time they are likely to go through a million dollars in

medical costs. Insurance companies have to wake up and realize that some cancers are curable. There are millions of survivors out there who are living long, healthy, and productive lives.

Advocacy doesn't necessarily mean you will change the system overnight. But it will give you a shot at getting your voice heard. And it just might give you some measure of power over your health care destiny. Ralph Nader asserts:

Advocacy can work if enough people believe in it. People *can* make a difference. Look at all the cancer survivors there are! If enough of them work together, they can make things happen. After all, look what the disabled were able to do on disability rights. The media aren't interested in reporting on closed-door advocacy. They like to see people out there marching and demanding change. The question is, when are you going to start?

Resources for Insurance Information

The following agencies and associations can provide you with further information on insurance questions.

AMERICAN COUNCIL OF LIFE INSURANCE
1001 Pennsylvania Avenue N.W.
Washington, DC 20004
(202) 624-2000

HEALTH INSURANCE ASSOCIATION OF AMERICA
1025 Connecticut Avenue N.W.
Washington, DC 20036
(202) 223-7780
Industry associations that represent commercial insurers.
Both organizations provide information to the public on
health, life, and disability insurance.

BLUE CROSS/BLUE SHIELD ASSOCIATIONS
233 North Michigan Avenue
Chicago, IL 60601
(312) 938-6000
Provides information on Blue Cross/Blue Shield coverage
offered in every state, including the availability of annual
open enrollment periods.

CHAMPAIGN COUNTY HEALTH CARE CONSUMERS
ORGANIZATION
44 Main Street, Suite 208
Champaign, IL 61820
(217) 352-6533
A nonprofit community-based organization dedicated to
promoting health care reform through consumer advocacy,
community education, and collective action on the part of
concerned citizens.

COMMUNICATING FOR AGRICULTURE, INC.
2626 East 82nd Street, Suite 325
Bloomington, MN 55425
(612) 854-9000
A national rural organization offering up-to-date information on high-risk insurance pools. Since 1975, Communicating for Agriculture has served as a strong advocate for the
establishment of these state-run risk pools.

MEDICAL INFORMATION BUREAU, INC. (MIB)
P.O. Box 105
Essex Station
Boston, MA 02112
(617) 426-3660
Write to the MIB to request a copy of your medical records
so that you can verify the information and correct any in-
accuracies. You may want to call the MIB first to find out the
type of information it needs (i.e., your date of birth, Social
Security number, etc.) to process your request.

THE NATIONAL CONSUMER HELPLINE
(800) 942-4242

NATIONAL INSURANCE CONSUMER ORGANIZATION (NICO)
121 North Payne Street
Alexandria, VA 22314
(703) 549-8050
NICO is a nonprofit public interest advocacy and education organization established in 1980 by Ralph Nader and Robert Hunter (former federal insurance administrator under Presidents Ford and Carter). NICO provides information on health and life insurance.

NATIONAL UNDERWRITERS COMPANY
420 East Fourth Street
Cincinnati, OH 45202
(513) 721-2140
Publishes the annual guide *Who Writes What in Life and Health Insurance*.

7

When the Résumé Includes Cancer

IN WESTERN SOCIETY, what you do for a living is a vital measure of who you are. Work is your public voice, a cultural I.D. tag. It is also an important source of security, self-esteem, and if you're lucky, happiness. Whether you toil for material rewards or personal fulfillment, power or prestige, work provides you with the chance to fulfill your ambitions and fix a course in life.

Most people value their right to work; it is essential to their economic and emotional well-being. With cancer survivors, it takes on added significance: going back to work means getting back to normal. But for some, there is an unexpected shock on returning to the job: discrimination. It might be blatant and overt, such as reduced company benefits, outright dismissal, or rejection of a job application. But more often it takes a quieter, subtler form. You may notice it in the hesitancy before a handshake, in the glances and whispers of co-workers, or in the promotions or pay hikes that never quite materialize. As a result, job opportunities, access to health insurance, even your self-esteem are jeopardized.

Cancer's Stigma in the Work Place

How prevalent is discrimination against cancer survivors? According to Barbara Hoffman, a New Jersey-based disability rights lawyer and co-author with Dr. Fitzhugh Mullan of *Charting the Journey: The Cancer Survivor's Almanac of Resources* (Consumer Reports, 1990), approximately 25 percent of all recovered cancer patients (roughly 1.25 million people) experience some form of employment discrimination. Several independent studies have shown the percentage to be even higher. Surveys conducted between 1976 and 1982 by Frances Feldman, a University of Southern California professor of social work, revealed that 54 percent of survivors in white-collar jobs and 84 percent in blue-collar positions were met with some form of discriminatory behavior when they returned to work. Recovered cancer patients reported problems ranging from ostracism by fellow employees and reduced health benefits to demotion and dismissal.

Even the fear of discrimination itself can be enough to diminish job opportunities. For instance, many survivors remain in undesirable or unfulfilling jobs because they worry — not without reason — that they will lose their group health benefits if they change companies. Some are even reluctant to take advantage of sick leave, fearing that by doing so their jobs may be jeopardized.

Employment discrimination can be especially difficult for young survivors who have little or no previous experience in the job market. Many find it is an uphill fight trying to prove that a cancer history is not an impediment to a productive career.

That was Alex's experience when he applied for a job with his hometown police force. Now thirty-two, Alex was in his last year of college when he was diagnosed with testicular cancer. After surgery and five weeks of radiation, he was told there was no further sign of malignancy.

Two years later, married and the father of two young sons, Alex decided to apply for a job as city police officer. "I was looking for the kind of job that would really push me. I wanted to be challenged, and at the same time have a positive impact on people's lives. The job of police officer seemed to fit the bill."

There was one hitch, however. After he applied for the job, Alex had to contend with a city policy governing the hiring of cancer survivors.

At the time I began preliminary test procedures with the police department, it never occurred to me that I might be rejected because of cancer. I signed up, took the first round of tests, and thought I was on my way. I was told that if my background information checked out, I'd be all set to start police academy classes.

The background check involved a medical history and exam. I filled out all the information and then took the physical. Never in my wildest dreams did I think that it would make a difference. Since my short bout with cancer two years earlier, I was as healthy as anyone can be. I'd been athletic enough to go out for both high school and college basketball, and I still played with a city team. My doctor said I had about as much chance of getting cancer as the next guy. The way I saw it, I was more likely to be killed in the line of duty than die of cancer.

So I was stunned when I received a police department form letter stating: "Reject. Testicular cancer. Must have five-year free period." I could only think that they had somehow made a mistake. They obviously didn't understand my situation.

I talked to my doctor about it, and he wrote a letter stating that my current health and prognosis were excellent. Using his letter, I appealed the decision. A month or two later I received the same form letter back rejecting me. I had one more chance to appeal.

This time, the police department arranged to have me examined by a local oncologist. I was optimistic about my chances, since I presumed this cancer specialist would know the score and explain to the department that I was fit to join the force.

I waited to hear, then waited some more. I finally went down to the police department and learned that my final appeal had also been rejected. It seems their decision was based on a municipal policy regarding the hiring of anyone with a history of cancer. It was an old law, and it didn't take into account different kinds of cancer.

At this point I was mad as hell. I knew I had to do something, not just for myself but for every survivor who might be faced with the same problem. So I talked to a hospital social worker who then suggested I contact the local office of the American Cancer Society [ACS]. They in turn provided me with a lot of information outlining my rights as a survivor. They informed me that the police department's policy was illegal. As it turned out, in my state, California, the Fair Employment and Housing Act strictly prohibits discrimination against cancer survivors. The city law that the police department had used to reject me was in fact a violation of state law.

The ACS referred me to the Employment Law Center, which is a project of the Legal Aid Society of San Francisco, and eventually one of their attorneys took my case. We sued the city police department and five years after my initial rejection, we settled the case out of court.

It was a long battle, but I feel I accomplished a lot. I was not only offered a job with the city police department, but I was given five years' seniority. I was also awarded back pay, compensatory damages, and attorneys' fees. What I'm most proud of, though, is that my case forced the city to change its discriminatory hiring policy so that it's no longer governed by an arbitrary five-year cure criterion. From now on, each case involving cancer must be decided on an individual basis.

Like Alex, you may have come away from your cancer experience with a compelling desire to give something back, to make a difference. Or perhaps you feel a need to "prove" your level of wellness. Alex was not about to let stereotypical thinking interfere with his career goals. He fought back and won. Now in his seventh year with a county police force, Alex was recently voted Most Valuable Officer of the Year by his peers.

The Myths Behind
Cancer-based Discrimination

Alex poses the question all survivors ask: If my doctor considers me cured, why shouldn't society?

The reason is clear: the medical community's view of cancer is based on a realistic understanding of the disease and greater optimism about its treatment. Social attitudes, however, remain tinged with irrational fear. But that's nothing new. For centuries, cancer has been the focus of myth and misunderstanding and the anchor for prejudice and discrimination. By the turn of this century, Americans had developed such a terrible phobia of the disease that few people dared even to whisper its name out loud.

The public's attitude has certainly evolved since then. But old ways of thinking die hard. Despite the progress made in diagnosis and treatment, cancer's reputation remains tethered to an assortment of punishing myths. Barbara Hoffman outlines three myths in particular that continue to influence the way some employers perceive survivors.

THE "DEATH SENTENCE" MYTH

This myth assumes that cancer is an inevitably fatal disease, and those who have it will die prematurely. Employers who buy into this way of thinking are reluctant to hire a cancer survivor. The result? You may want to formulate long-term career plans, but your employer has you pegged for a short-term life.

Belief in this myth stems chiefly from ignorance. For example, most people are surprised to learn that cancer accounts for just 20 percent of deaths in the United States, whereas cardiovascular disease kills twice as many people. In fact, cancer is now considered *the most curable* of serious chronic diseases. The National Cancer Institute reports that more than half of all people diagnosed with cancer today will survive their illness and go on to lead full, productive lives. The current cure rate has increased significantly from just thirty years ago, when the figure hovered around 30 percent. Survival rates for young adult and childhood cancers are particularly impressive, with rates as high as 80 and 90 percent.

THE "UNPRODUCTIVE WORKER" MYTH

Employers often worry that survivors won't be able to do their fair share of work or will need assistance performing their jobs. Some also suspect that turnover and absentee rates will be higher for those with a cancer history.

This myth was dispelled years ago by two landmark studies. The first of these was conducted by the Metropolitan Life Insurance Company. From 1959 to 1972, Metropolitan tracked the employment records of seventy-four survivors and found no difference in absenteeism, turnover, or work performance from those of nonsurvivor employees. According to their findings, not one survivor had been dismissed as a result of poor performance. The results were so encouraging that the study concluded that the hiring of cancer survivors was "sound industrial practice."

In 1972, a study by the American Telephone and Telegraph Company revealed that approximately 80 percent of 1,351 AT&T employees diagnosed with cancer returned to their jobs after completion of treatment. The study concluded that a cancer diagnosis did not automatically shorten or subvert an employee's productive life.

What ultimately makes the unproductive worker myth so

ironic is that survivors often feel that their cancer experience has made them more appreciative of life and therefore better workers. They have emerged from treatment confident in their ability to handle the challenges of a demanding job. As Alex says: "I think cancer made me a better cop. You don't know what facing danger is until you've had to fight a life-threatening disease. It has also given me a greater sense of compassion and understanding of other people."

THE "CANCER IS CONTAGIOUS" MYTH

The persistence of this myth is testament to how deeply in-grained cancerphobia remains in our culture. Cancer is no more contagious than arthritis or poor vision. Still, some people act as though it is, in effect socially quarantining the survivor.

I recently heard from a survivor who was fired from his job as a restaurant chef because it was feared he might contami-nate the food. A woman I know was asked during a job inter-view if she had ever been seriously ill. When she answered that she was a survivor of childhood leukemia, her inter-viewer asked, "How did you catch that?"

How does this myth endure amid today's barrage of media coverage on cancer? Clearly some people cling to cancer mythology the way others cling to superstitious thinking. They may have heard cancer isn't contagious, but they aren't taking any chances.

You, Your Employer, and the Law

Before moving any further into this chapter, you should know where you stand legally on the issue of employment discrimination. Whether you have a job or are looking for one, keep in mind that discrimination based on a history of cancer is a violation of federal law, and may also be in violation of local state law. A clear understanding of your legal rights can foster the self-confidence you need to stand up to discriminatory practices.

FEDERAL LAWS

The Rehabilitation Act of 1973. This law, amended in 1978 and 1984, prohibits discrimination against the disabled by employers who receive federal funding or federal contracts of more than $2,500 annually. The law also protects federal employees. Because the Rehabilitation Act extends only to a limited number of employers, it falls short of offering all survivors a legal remedy to work-related discrimination.

Survivors should be aware of three key parts of the Rehabilitation Act: Sections 501, 503, and 504. Sections 501 and 503 protect disabled people from employment discrimination by federal agencies and federal contractors. These employers are also required to take affirmative action to hire, place, and advance disabled people.

Section 504 of the act protects against discrimination in all federally assisted programs and activities (including hospitals, schools, and colleges). Section 504 states that

No otherwise qualified handicapped individual in the United States . . . shall, solely by reason of his handicap, be excluded from participation in, be denied the benefits of, or be subjected to discrimination under any program or activity receiving Federal financial assistance.

Section 7(7) of the act defines a "handicapped individual" as "any person who (i) has a physical or mental impairment which substantially limits one or more of such person's major life activities, (ii) has a record of such an impairment, or (iii) is regarded as having such an impairment." This broad definition includes people who may not consider themselves handicapped or disabled, including many cancer survivors. Although the act does not specifically list cancer as a disability, the U.S. Supreme Court has determined that cancer is covered under this law.

The Rehabilitation Act prohibits covered employers from discrimination in hiring, promotions, transfers, wages and salaries, benefits (including health and life insurance), and termination. Under the act, a covered employer cannot require an applicant to undergo a medical or physical examination prior to offering that person a job. Once an applicant has been offered a job, however, a medical history or exam may be required, but only if it is required of other applicants. In addition, employers are required to provide "reasonable accommodation" to disabled employees (more on this later in the chapter).

Survivors who take legal action under Sections 501 and 504 of the act can file for job reinstatement, attorneys' fees, injunctive relief (to halt the discriminatory practice), and back pay. Employers who violate the law risk having their federal funds withheld, including cancellation of any federal contracts. Sections 503 and 504 of the Rehabilitation Act of 1973 are handled by separate government offices (see listings at the end of this chapter).

If you decide to file a complaint under this law, remember to

• *File your claim promptly.* Federal employees or applicants to federal jobs must notify the equal employment opportunity office of the agency that took discriminatory action within thirty days of the action. Employees and applicants of employers who have federal contracts or subcontracts must notify the U.S. Department of Labor within 180 days of a discriminatory act. *If you miss the deadline, your claim may be ruled*

invalid. You must also file with the agency that administers federal funding to the employer within 180 days.
• *Document your claim.* When filing your claim, be as specific as you can about the discriminatory action. A complete and detailed statement will help speed along the investigation of your complaint. Get the facts down in writing and keep photocopies of any paperwork or correspondence. Also, be sure to compile as much documentation as you can, including medical records, supporting letters from doctors, and favorable statements from coworkers and supervisors.

The Americans with Disabilities Act of 1990 (ADA). This landmark legislation picks up where the federal Rehabilitation Act left off by protecting the employment rights of disabled people in the private sector. Hailed by President Bush as "the world's first declaration of equality for people with disabilities," the ADA guarantees equal rights in the work place as well as equal access to public facilities to the approximately forty-three million disabled Americans (including cancer patients and survivors).

This wide-ranging civil rights bill makes it illegal for an employer to discriminate against a qualified applicant or employee who is disabled, has a history of a disability, or is perceived as having a disability. It also forbids discrimination against disabled people in all public services (such as state and local government offices), public accommodations (hotels, restaurants, shopping centers, and so on), transportation, and telecommunication.

The ADA states that employers must provide reasonable accommodation to qualified disabled employees. The act contains the same broad definition of "disability" put forth in Section 504 of the Rehabilitation Act of 1973. Employers are also prohibited from asking medical questions before offering applicants a job unless their health history has strict bearing on work performance. Nor can applicants be required to undergo a preemployment medical exam unless it is (1) job related, and (2) requested of all employees.

It is important to note that the ADA's employment discrimination provisions will not take effect until July 26, 1992, when coverage will extend to private businesses with twenty-five or more employees. After July 26, 1994, coverage will be further extended to companies with fifteen or more employees. In other words, if you work for or apply to a company that employs only twelve people and you encounter discrimination, ADA won't be of much help. Instead you will have to rely on the strength of your state's disability laws or, if appropriate, the Rehabilitation Act of 1973.

Under the ADA, survivors may seek remedies against employers who violate the law, including injunctive relief and back pay, if they are denied a job or fired as a result of their disability. Once the ADA takes effect in 1992, it will be enforced by the U.S. Equal Employment Opportunity Commission (EEOC). If you plan to take action against an employer, call the EEOC and find out what procedures you need to follow in order to file a complaint under the ADA. For more information about your rights under this law, call the EEOC's Public Information Office at (800) 872-3362.

STATE LAWS

In addition to these federal statutes, forty-five states and the District of Columbia have laws proscribing employment discrimination against the disabled. The amount and type of protection available vary from state to state. However, three states — California, Vermont, and New Mexico — have laws that expressly prohibit discrimination based on a cancer history. The California Fair Employment and Housing Act (FEHA), for instance, prohibits employment discrimination based on a "medical condition" or "physical handicap." The "medical condition" defined in FEHA refers to "any health impairment related to or associated with a diagnosis of cancer, for which a person has been rehabilitated or cured, based on competent medical evidence." The law covers all California businesses employing five or more people.

To find out what the laws are in your state, contact the state agency that enforces employment rights, your local bar association, a chapter of the American Cancer Society, or cancer support groups that offer employment-related resources. They can help you find out how to file a complaint and what the deadlines are for filing.

How to Deal with Work Place Discrimination

Now that you have an understanding of both the myths that provoke employment discrimination and the laws that prohibit it, you should be aware of how both can affect your return to the work force or your entry into it. Your own attitude and behavior also play an important part in how well you finesse an encounter with cancer-based discrimination.

DISCRIMINATORY HIRING PRACTICES

A number of Cancervive members have related stories of how they were hired for a position only to be rejected after a preemployment physical exam revealed their history of cancer. Others were required to answer health questions during their interview, and an honest answer almost always cost them the job.

I've mentioned it before, but it bears repeating: unless you have specific physical or mental limitations that affect work-related activities, your cancer history should have no bearing on your job qualifications. In short, an employer cannot refuse to hire you solely on the basis of your medical history.

Although the ADA guarantees this, its provision banning discriminatory hiring will not take effect until 1992. Until then you must rely on state law, or if the company to which you are applying is federally funded, the Rehabilitation Act. Employers in states governed by disability rights laws may ask only job-related questions. The focus of an employer's questions should be whether you can perform the job; the employer cannot question you generally about your disability.

Even with these laws in place, however, don't expect discriminatory hiring practices to disappear anytime soon. As health care costs and insurance premiums maintain their upward spiral, employers will continue to look for loopholes in the law. It is over this bottom-line issue that your interests and those of an employer are most likely to collide.

Although health benefits are usually extended to employees who return to their jobs after cancer treatment, insurers will as a matter of course raise a company's premium once an employee has been diagnosed with cancer or is known to have had the disease. Consequently, employers are often reluctant to hire anyone with a serious preexisting medical condition, fearful that their insurance rates will skyrocket. This is a particular problem for smaller businesses, which, unlike large corporations, don't have a large pool of employees or the budget to absorb higher insurance rates. As a result, many smaller firms are forced to choose between affordable insurance coverage and the welfare of an employee with a cancer history.

Until insurance companies are required to liberalize their policies regarding preexisting conditions, or until the United States implements a program of national health insurance, this issue will remain an employer's strongest argument against hiring cancer survivors. For further information on work-based insurance problems, see Chapter 6.

SUGGESTIONS FOR JOB INTERVIEWS

Job interviews are stressful enough, but when you're worried about how your health history will influence your chances, they can be particularly nerve-racking. Even with an enlightened employer, it's not easy explaining cancer-related gaps in a résumé. An understanding of your rights can help you know what to do if and when you run into illegal pre-employment screening. When interviewing for a job, keep in mind these points:

* *Don't discriminate against yourself.* Unless you are directly asked, do not volunteer your cancer history to a prospective employer. But if you are asked, answer in a straightforward manner. If you lie and are later found out, the revelation could be grounds for dismissal.

  Ellen Daly serves as acting director of public affairs for the President's Committee on Employment of People with Disabilities in Washington, D.C. She suggests that if you are explicitly asked about cancer you should answer honestly and succinctly, stating that although you were treated for cancer in the past, you are now recovered and capable of doing the job. She adds:

  Should you have any visible handicaps secondary to your cancer, find an opportunity during the interview to discuss your disability with the employer, if only to assure him or her that you are capable of doing the job. This also gives you a chance to alleviate the employer's fears and answer questions regarding any possible on-the-job accommodations that your handicap may require.

  But above all, be positive and assertive. Impress upon the employer your capabilities and strengths. Don't hesitate to say at the end of the interview, "I want this job, and this is how I intend to carry out the responsibilities involved." That can really impress an employer.

Some survivors have an overriding need to explain their cancer history to a potential employer. That can be a mistake. An employer is only interested in one issue: can you do the job? Don't forget that your role during a job interview is that of salesperson. What you are selling is your ability to help the employer run the business as effectively as possible, so conduct the interview on those terms. As Barbara Hoffman says, "You have no moral or legal obligation to talk about your cancer unless it has some bearing on job performance. After all, you're looking for a job, not approval."

An equally important point: try not to appear overly concerned about the type of insurance coverage or benefits package offered. Your potential boss wants you to be first and foremost interested in the job. Once you've been officially offered the position, then by all means look into benefits.

• *Get your doctor's endorsement.* An employee's physical limitations are obviously going to be a concern to any employer. If a potential employer has questions or doubts about your ability to perform the job, ask your employer to contact your doctor (or better yet, bring a letter from your doctor to the interview). Everyone likes to be reassured by experts, and a call or letter from your physician will give your application a medical "seal of approval." Many survivors have found this strategy to be very effective.

• *Know your legal rights.* Don't forget that even though you may have no discernible handicap, laws providing help for disabled individuals also apply to cancer patients and survivors. Whether or not you consider yourself disabled, that's where your protection lies under the law.

• *Physical examinations are at times a condition of hiring.* In some instances, a medical history or physical exam is an essential part of determining whether a person is appropriate for a particular job. In Alex's case, law enforcement departments called for all applicants to be screened for any medical conditions or impairments that could create on-the-job problems. If physical fitness is a requirement for the position — as it would be for any job where the public's health and safety is at stake — then medical screening would be appropriate.

• *Don't give in to discrimination.* If, during or after a job interview, you suspect that an employer has engaged in discriminatory practices, you have the right to take action. You can do this first by letting your interviewer know, in a calm and diplomatic way, that you are aware of the laws protecting cancer survivors. Don't be confrontational. Simply bring it to the employer's attention that you intend to pursue the matter further. You may then want to contact your local branch of the American Cancer Society to determine how to proceed.

DISCRIMINATORY PRACTICES ON THE JOB

Employment discrimination is by no means limited to hiring practices. More often it happens on the job, where the overt or covert prejudicial attitudes of employers and coworkers can result in biased behavior. For instance, you may have returned to work to find that your job duties have been curtailed or that you've been transferred, against your wishes, to a less desirable branch office or location. Or perhaps your request for a promotion or entry into an advanced training program was denied. A career curve ball is not necessarily a discriminatory action, however. Many other factors can come into play, such as office politics, seniority, the company's bottom line, your own work performance and attitude, even the state of the economy. As a result, employment discrimination inhabits a very gray legal area.

Michael Spekter is an attorney specializing in employment

law in Washington, D.C., who is also an eleven-year survivor of Hodgkin's disease. He has represented many survivors who have faced cancer-based discrimination in the work place.

It isn't easy to define what constitutes employment discrimination, let alone try to prove it. That is one reason why more survivors haven't initiated lawsuits. It appears that the only successful cases are those where there is either a clear verbal or paper trail of blatant discrimination.

But let's assume that you are performing your job satisfactorily and you are still passed over for that long-awaited promotion. How can you determine whether or not the action is discriminatory?

Begin by taking a cold, hard look at the situation. Try to understand exactly what has happened. Can you say with absolute certainty that cancer played a part in it? Some survivors are quick to interpret denial of a promotion, a demotion, or an undesirable transfer as evidence of cancer-based discrimination. They allow themselves to fall into the "victim" trap, where every slight is perceived to be a sure sign of prejudice.

It's easy to misinterpret a ruthless yet legitimate business decision as a discriminatory action — especially if that decision is contrary to your wishes or expectations. Try to depersonalize the situation and determine what else might have influenced it.

By all means, don't rule out your own attitude and orientation toward work. It could be that cancer has altered your priorities, and the driving ambition you once had for your job has now shifted to other means of self-fulfillment. Such a change could in itself greatly influence the speed and direction of your career.

It is also possible that cancer has had a deleterious effect on your self-esteem. You may no longer feel capable of competing with "healthy" coworkers. That kind of self-doubt is going to hold you back more than any physical disability or discriminatory action. Remember that confidence is contagious. If you have faith in your abilities, chances are others will too.

If, however, after weighing the situation, you are convinced that discriminatory behavior is at the root of your problem, you may want to do something about it. The information provided below is not intended as legal advice, but rather as suggestions on how you might resolve a perceived discriminatory action.

- *Determine how you want to handle it.* Do you think your employer would be open to resolving the situation? If so, you may want to work through your problem internally, either by dealing directly with your supervisor, personnel director, or union representative or by taking advantage of whatever administrative complaint procedure your company offers employees. If not, you may find it necessary to file a formal complaint with an administrative agency outside the company. Try to determine what would be the most effective — and least frustrating — way to resolve the situation.
- *Document your claim.* Be sure to keep a record of any action you perceive to be discriminatory. This record will be helpful later on if you decide to take legal action. Remember to include details of the incident such as the date, the time, and the names of people involved — including any coworkers who happen to have witnessed it.
- *Research your rights under the law.* Familiarize yourself with both state and federal laws protecting the on-the-job rights of disabled people. Find out where you stand and if your problem can be defined as discriminatory. Be aware that

many disability laws require that you contact specific administrative agencies before you take legal action. Also, determine what the deadlines are for applying. If you overlook or in some way fail to comply with these administrative procedures, your claim could be invalidated.

• *Get advice.* If you still haven't been able to resolve your grievance, you may want to consult with an employment rights agency or nonprofit advocacy group in your community. These organizations can help you sort out your legal rights and refer you to other resources.

• *Get a lawyer.* If you have the funds and fortitude, you may choose to retain a lawyer, preferably one who specializes in employment law. If you can't afford to hire an attorney, call your local bar association. It may be able to refer you to a legal aid lawyer at little or no cost.

However you handle your situation, know that you have a right not to be discriminated against because of your cancer history. A caveat: one of the reasons on-the-job discrimination can be so difficult to identify is that an employer's prejudicial attitudes are often cloaked in concern and solicitude. My own experience revealed just how subtle this kind of discrimination can be. At the beginning of this book, I described how I was once up for promotion with a large cosmetics firm. I lost out when a coworker suggested to the company's vice president that my cancer history might interfere with my ability to do the job. It was later explained to me that I had been "spared" the promotion because it was thought that the extensive travel required would be too strenuous for me.

Few things are as infuriating as someone deciding the fate of your career for you. It's even more maddening when your employer does it "for your own good." No one has the right to prevent you from fulfilling your ambitions and enacting career decisions. Of course, it's important that you know your limitations and what you can realistically achieve. But with the Americans with Disabilities Act, you have greater opportunity to fight back if office prejudice is interfering with your ambitions.

Office Ostracism. One work place worry that plagues survivors is determining how to deal with the insensitive or inappropriate responses of coworkers. Although the public is far less cancerphobic than it once was, I still hear from survivors who were shunned at work or subject to hostile remarks. Fear of contagion appears to be the underlying reason for a good deal of office prejudice. A somewhat bizarre example of such discrimination is the experience of a survivor named Veronica, forty-four, who took time off from her job as an administrative assistant at a manufacturing firm to undergo treatment for cervical cancer. Her first day back at work was, as she describes it, a rather "sticky" affair.

Thank God for Pap smears. It caught my cancer in its earliest stage. Three weeks after the operation, I headed right back to work. The morning of my return I found a big bouquet of flowers sitting on my desk. Everyone at the office was terrific — very friendly and helpful. As a "welcome back" gesture, several coworkers announced that they wanted to treat me to lunch. I was beginning to feel like queen for a day.

As it turned out, not everyone was thrilled to have me back. After I returned from lunch, I grabbed a cup of coffee and sat down at my desk. Right away I noticed something was wrong; the desk was damp and slightly sticky. It also smelled funny. I picked up the phone and noticed that it was sticky too. So were the files, my pens and pencils, the computer — everything on and around my desk had a slight film of *something* on it.

I immediately asked my boss about it. At first she thought I was joking, but once she sat down at my desk she was as baffled as I was. I asked around and no one would give me a satisfactory answer. I decided to check with my friend Tom. He looked so sheepish, I could tell right away that he knew. I badgered him a bit and he finally told me that a couple of the secretaries sitting near me had decided to disinfect my entire office with Lysol — just in case what I had was catching.

Veronica approached her boss, explained what had happened, and asked for suggestions on how to handle it. Together they decided to organize an informal "cancer conference." The following morning, a memo was issued to all office personnel. Everyone was asked to grab a cup of coffee and take a seat in the conference room.

Veronica's boss supplied the doughnuts and Veronica supplied the facts, talking about her recent illness as she handed out pamphlets on cervical cancer.

I provided all the details, making it very clear that cancer was in no way a communicable disease. I didn't name names and I didn't get angry. I simply stated that I thought they might have questions about what had happened to me, and that this was the best way to handle it. I told them that except for the loss of my uterus, I was the same old Veronica.

Even though most of my coworkers were already fairly knowledgeable about cancer, I could tell that the discussion really made an impact, and not just on the Lysol squad. I think it put everyone at ease hearing me talk openly about my experience and seeing the information in black and white. It gave me a chance to answer all the unspoken questions they'd been too embarrassed or afraid to ask. It wasn't exactly the easiest thing I've ever done, but the results were worth it.

No one enjoys being on the receiving end of office gossip or discriminatory behavior. Nor should you be expected to put up with it. Your best method of combating it is through information and education. Should you encounter office prejudice, consider the following:

• *Check your own attitude.* Are your coworkers treating you differently since you've returned, or are they merely reacting to the signals you're giving out? It's not unusual for survivors to have mixed feelings about what they want out of life after cancer. Look inside yourself before you misinterpret the actions and attitudes of others. Consider whether or not the problem is due to your own difficulty in readjusting to the work place.

- *Talk to the boss.* It is the responsibility of your boss or office supervisor to ensure that the office runs smoothly and the environment promotes productivity. If a coworker's prejudicial actions are interfering with your ability to get the job done, ask your boss to act as intermediary.

- *Organize an office meeting.* This approach worked for Veronica, as it has for several other Cancervive members. (Be sure to clear it with your boss or supervisor first.) Also, consider distributing pamphlets or articles that deal with the kind of cancer you had. Both the American Cancer Society and the National Cancer Institute publish material that explain the facts in easy-to-read terms. If you can arrange it, invite a social worker or nurse from your hospital to speak to the group.

You may discover, as Veronica did, that the easiest way to squelch office fear and prejudice is to be as candid as you can about your cancer experience. Of course, that doesn't mean you need to bare your soul and reveal personal details. Instead, emphasize whatever positive views you've gained from the experience. For the one or two individuals in your office who may still cling stubbornly to the myths about cancer, a clear insight into your illness might be just the thing to change their minds.

If your illness has resulted in physical impairments, fellow employees will no doubt be uncertain of how to respond to you. Take the initiative and break the ice — and don't forget the power of laughter. After all, one of the easiest ways to disarm people is to make them laugh. If you can accept your disability, even laugh about it, why shouldn't your coworkers? Veronica offers an example of how a sense of humor can put others at ease:

> One of the men in my office didn't know what to say to me. He seemed so uptight and embarrassed. Then one day I mentioned to him that thanks to my hysterectomy I was saving a bundle on contraceptives. We both had a good laugh, and now he's not half as nervous around me as he used to be.

• *Consider filing a formal complaint.* As a last resort, you may want to consider taking legal action — but only as a last resort. Keep in mind that proving office harassment is very tricky. Also, if you are at all interested in keeping your job and maintaining friendships with coworkers, filing a lawsuit is probably not the way to go. Says Barbara Hoffman:

> We all tend to forget that there's no law out there that says people can't be jerks. A coworker's action has to be pretty blatant before you should even consider talking to a lawyer. By blatant I mean any action or behavior that impedes your ability to get the job done. In most instances, diplomacy and goodwill work a lot better than formal complaints and lawsuits. However, if after trying all other options, a coworker is continuing to make your work life impossible, this may be the only way to resolve it.

Vocational Rehabilitation

Although most survivors are physically able to return to work, some find that cancer has caused permanent changes or restrictions that limit their former capabilities. If either a physical or a mental impairment has made it difficult for you to return to your job, consider redirecting your talents and skills through job retraining. Help is available through your state-run Vocational Rehabilitation Administration.

Recovering cancer patients often assume that vocational

rehabilitation is limited to people with obvious impairments, such as amputees or persons who have had laryngectomies. It isn't. Cancer treatment can also result in impairments such as loss of hearing, agility, or strength which can directly affect your ability to resume your former line of work. Others undergo subtler, less perceptible changes. Survivors of brain cancer, for example, often have no outward signs of impairment yet may struggle with memory loss, motor skill problems, and cognitive functioning. Total rehabilitation — physical, psychosocial, and vocational — is essential to every cancer patient's recovery. Regardless of your disability, the objective is to get your life and career goals back on track.

Tim is a survivor who took advantage of a rehabilitation program to redirect his career after cancer. The twenty-eight-year-old aspiring journalist recently described how he was fired from his job after a bout with soft-tissue cancer.

I developed a tumor in my abdominal cavity two years ago. At the time I was working at a supermarket, stocking shelves at night. When I told my supervisor about the diagnosis, he suggested that I take a leave of absence until I was finished with treatment. My cancer was stage three and so I got the whole nine yards: surgery, chemo, and radiation. I needed every day of my six-month medical leave to get through it all.

Two days after I returned to work, I knew I still wasn't up to par. I discovered that I could no longer do the heavy lifting that the job required. During surgery the doctors had removed some of my abdominal muscles, which made lifting heavy objects nearly impossible. That caused problems at work, since my store's employment policy required all employees to be capable of performing every store duty, from manning the cash register to stocking shelves.

My supervisor noticed the difficulty I was having and suggested I take more time off to recuperate. But I didn't want that. I was eager to work; it gave me the feeling that I was back in control of my life. I asked if I could be assigned to another position, something that wouldn't require a lot of lifting. My supervisor said it wasn't possible; to do so would mean bumping another employee out of his position. So instead, I was fired.

They told me the reason I was let go was because I'd used up all my medical leave. But I think they just didn't want the bother of retraining me; it was easier to replace me. I also heard through the grapevine that my supervisor was worried I might injure myself on the job or get sick again.

I think it was definitely a discriminatory move, but at that point I knew I'd have a tough time proving it. Still, I was both able and eager to work for the company in some other capacity. I had lots of experience working for other grocery stores, doing everything from checking to management. But they insisted on hanging me up on store "policy." That really got me mad, because I know that several of the little old ladies working cashier have never been asked to stock shelves.

In a way, though, it all turned out for the best. I have a college degree in communications, and I'd been wanting to get into a more challenging career. This gave me the shove I needed. During one of my checkups, my doctor suggested I look into vocational rehabilitation. So for the last six months I've been training with a local VR program for a new career in journalism. I have to say, getting fired wasn't much fun, but it certainly helped point me in the right direction.

Most work-able survivors have no difficulty returning to their jobs, and some find that their employers are supportive of their needs as recovering patients. But as Tim's story illustrates, even survivors with minimum dysfunction can encounter problems if their employers are unwilling or unable to accommodate them. You may have experienced a similar situation. You want to work, but now that your old job is no longer appropriate for you, your employer isn't sure what to do. You suggest retraining. Your boss suggests you look for another job. What options are available to you?

The first strategy you should pursue is to determine your job rights. Under the law your employer may be obliged to provide you with "reasonable accommodation," which means that the company must take steps to accommodate a disabled person's special needs. Reasonable accommodation might include modifying a work environment (for instance, to accommodate an employee's wheelchair), restructuring the job, modifying work schedules, reassigning duties, or installing special devices (such as telephones for the hearing-impaired).

But there is a catch. Employers are not required to provide accommodation if they can demonstrate that it would result in "undue hardship." Barbara Hoffman points out that the definition of what constitutes undue hardship is fuzzy and includes consideration of several factors, such as the size of the business, the cost and nature of the accommodation in question, and the number of employees who would be affected by the accommodation.

It depends on the particulars of each case. In a large corporation, for example, it might not be a hardship to relocate or retrain a disabled employee, even if it means shuffling around the work schedules of several coworkers. However, this could very well create a lot of disruption for a small business and therefore be considered an undue burden. In short, if your employer can prove that to retrain you or accommodate you in some other capacity would be too burdensome for the company, you could be out of luck — and out of a job.

There are other options. But before you go any further, you need to acknowledge your disability and accept that it has resulted in a vocational handicap. That may sound all too obvious, but the reality is that many survivors subject themselves to the pain of repeated job rejection simply because they are reluctant to admit their handicap. They've allowed denial to interfere with their rehabilitation.

Then again, some survivors paint themselves into a different corner. They have no trouble accepting their disability; in fact, they've not only acknowledged it, they've allowed it to dominate their lives. These survivors often conclude that as a result of their handicap their productivity is kaput, and therefore their work life is over.

If this is happening to you, it's very possible that your self-esteem and self-image are in need of rehabilitation as well. By all means, don't overlook this aspect of "retraining" yourself for the work place through either private therapy or a support group. Take stock of your vocational skills and career goals. Even if cancer has severely impaired your former work abilities, remember that you still have much to offer the world. Ask yourself how you might transform your disability into an asset. As a survivor, you bring to any job a unique store of experience, strength, and understanding that most other people lack. But it's up to you to tap into this special reserve and then promote it.

You may find it helpful to discuss your needs with a professional. An occupational therapist can provide vocational guidance and discuss with you the kind of work you want to pursue as well as the programs that can best prepare you for a new job or career. Financial support during your rehabilitation is also an important concern and should be discussed with family members.

If you feel that you would benefit from vocational rehabilitation, your doctor or a hospital social worker can refer you to a local vocational rehabilitation or community service office. But don't feel you need a doctor's recommendation to get the ball rolling. Take the initiative and find out what you need to know about qualifying for local rehabilitation programs. To be eligible, it is generally required that you have both the capability and desire to return to the work force. Any disability that interferes with your normal line of work can qualify you for vocational rehabilitation assistance in the form of counseling, job training, financial assistance, or training in the use of special equipment. Vocational rehabilitation also provides special programs such as speech lessons for laryngectomy patients.

Every state is mandated to offer vocational rehabilitation programs. Specific qualifications vary from state to state, although survivors who qualify for Social Security disability automatically qualify for such programs. Call your state rehabilitation department (listed in the state government section of your phone directory) for further information about requirements.

Turning the Tide

For survivors who have encountered it, employment discrimination is one of the most frustrating and infuriating obstacles to life after cancer. Alex says he still feels tremendous anger over the issue of cancer-based discrimination, despite his victory over the police department's hiring policy.

There are really two battles you have to wage when you get cancer. First you fight the disease. Then you have to fight the biased attitudes and fears of employers and coworkers. I don't consider my cancer history to be a handicap, yet that's how it is perceived by some people.

I'm not saying survivors should get preferential treatment. But I do think we should have the same chance as everyone else. That's really all any survivor asks. And that's why I fought back.

If you experience work-related problems as a result of your cancer history, know that the law is on your side. But don't forget that current laws like the Americans with Disabilities Act provide protection, not a panacea. They are the tools recovered cancer patients have to empower themselves and enforce their rights in the work place. For survivors like Alex, that sometimes requires a trip to court. For others, like Veronica, it means fighting back on a more personal level with education and information.

My own encounter with job discrimination would have undoubtedly fared better if I had been more aware at the time of the legal remedies available to me. Since then I've learned the importance of advocacy. Had I known then what I know now, I most certainly would have fought for my employment rights. Instead I decided to start my own nonprofit organization. Now, I often joke to people, no one can fire me.

Happily, since I began Cancervive I've noticed a perceptible change in the public's attitude regarding cancer. Although much still needs to be done, both public and professional education is slowly chipping away at all the old myths. Organizations like the Employment Law Center, the American Cancer Society, the National Coalition for Cancer Survivorship, and Cancervive continue to advocate and advance the rights of patients and survivors.

But perhaps the most significant influence on public perception can be found in the growing ranks of survivors. Scores of prominent personalities — actors, politicians, sports figures — are beating the disease and demonstrating in full light of the media that a cancer history is not incompatible with a vital, productive career. Employers need only to remember that the highest office in the land was at one time held by a cancer survivor. To be sure, both Ronald Reagan (diagnosed with colon cancer in 1985) and his wife, Nancy (who underwent a mastectomy in 1987), made rapid returns to their busy schedules. Since leaving the White House, both have continued to lead active lives.

But although the tide is turning, the battle against cancer-based discrimination has yet to be won. Michael Spekter notes:

I've seen a significant decline in this kind of discrimination in the past decade, and I think the Americans with Disabilities Act is a culmination of this change in attitude. The A.D.A. is a terrific example of what disabled people can do when they join forces and advocate for an end to discrimination in the work place.

But even with tough laws on the books, prejudicial thinking isn't going to vanish overnight. Survivors will still have to find their way in a world that has yet to comprehend the full cancer picture.

That picture promises to keep improving. It is estimated that by the year 2000, one in every thousand adults will have survived some form of childhood cancer. As survival rates continue to rise, many more people will come to know first-hand what it means to beat cancer. They will realize, as you do, what it takes to face that challenge, and what the experience inexorably imparts to survivors. Perhaps that's when the last vestiges of fear will give way to appreciation and understanding.

Where to Go for Advice or Assistance

The agencies and organizations listed below can provide you with additional information about employment discrimination and other work-related issues.

For complaints under Section 503 of the federal Rehabilitation Act, contact

OFFICE OF FEDERAL CONTRACT COMPLIANCE PROGRAMS
U.S. Department of Labor
200 Constitution Avenue N.W., Room C-3325
Washington, DC 20210
(202) 523-9410

For complaints under Section 504 of the federal Rehabilitation Act, contact

DEPARTMENT OF HEALTH AND HUMAN SERVICES
200 Independence Avenue S.W.
Washington, DC 20201
(202) 619-0257

For information about the Americans with Disabilities Act, contact

U.S. EQUAL EMPLOYMENT OPPORTUNITY COMMISSION
1801 L Street N.W.
Washington, DC 20507
(800) 872-3362

AMERICAN CIVIL LIBERTIES UNION (ACLU)
132 West 43rd Street
New York, NY 10036
(212) 944-9800 (or call local listings)
Provides legal assistance for victims of discrimination.

CANDLELIGHTERS CHILDHOOD CANCER FOUNDATION
1901 Pennsylvania Avenue N.W., Suite 1001
Washington, DC 20006
(202) 659-5136
An international nonprofit organization formed by parents of young cancer patients. The founder of Candlelighters, Grace Monaco, is a leading advocate of survivors' rights in the work place.

DISABILITY RIGHTS CENTER
1346 Connecticut Avenue N.W.
Washington, DC 20036
(202) 223-3304

THE JOB ACCOMMODATION NETWORK
(800) 526-7234
A project of the President's Committee on the Employment of People with Disabilities, this hotline provides information regarding reasonable accommodation.

NATIONAL COALITION FOR CANCER SURVIVORSHIP
323 Eighth Street S.W.
Albuquerque, NM 87102
(505) 764-9956

A national network of individuals and organizations joined in the support and advocacy of survivorship concerns, including cancer-based discrimination.

NATIONAL REHABILITATION INFORMATION CENTER
   (NARIC)
U.S. Department of Education
National Institute on Disability Rehabilitation Research
8455 Colesville Road, Suite 935
Silver Spring, MD 20910
(800) 34-NARIC (voice/TDD)
A comprehensive, up-to-date information center and clearing-house providing resources and services for disabled people.

PRESIDENT'S COMMITTEE ON THE EMPLOYMENT OF
   PEOPLE WITH DISABILITIES
1111 20th Street N.W.
Washington, DC 20036
(202) 653-5044
A public-private partnership of individuals and organizations working together to improve the lives and employment opportunities of disabled people.

REHABILITATION SERVICES ADMINISTRATION
Department of Human Services
605 G Street N.W.
Washington, DC 20001
(202) 727-3211
Call for general information on vocational rehabilitation programs in your city, or check your telephone directory under state government listings for your state rehabilitation department.

8

The Double-Edged Sword: Long-Term Effects of Treatment

It is for science not only to add years to life, but more important, to add life to the years.

— Patricia A. Downie, *Cancer Rehabilitation*

CANCER TREATMENT keeps people alive, but often with undesirable consequences. Most of the unpleasant side effects associated with chemotherapy and radiation eventually subside once treatment ends. But some effects aren't as quick to fade, and others may unexpectedly crop up months or years later.

Until recently, attention to the long-term and late effects* of cancer treatment wasn't an issue for the medical community simply because most patients didn't live long enough. But the growing number of survivors is modifying that view. On-

---

* *Long-term effects* refers to the side effects that persist after treatment ends. *Late effects* are those that occur months or years later.

cologists, focused for so long on developing effective therapies to combat cancer, are beginning to take into account the full effect treatment has on the lives they have helped to extend.

Because some of the greatest increases in survival rates have been in patients with childhood cancers, most research on long-term effects has focused on young survivors. How cancer therapy has affected the adult survivor population remains largely unexamined territory.

Pyrrhic Victories

Twenty years ago, the chief issue facing cancer patients was survival; today, quality of life is equally important. Advances in treatment are eradicating many forms of malignancy which were once considered incurable, and this year hundreds of thousands of patients will leave the hospital with their lives rekindled. But for some recovered patients, the victory over cancer is in many ways a pyrrhic one. It is not unusual to hear these survivors describe cancer treatment as a double-edged sword, a weapon that damages the patient as it destroys the disease. Cancer treatment leaves them struggling with a variety of disabilities, from chronic pain and disfigurement to organ failure and memory loss. For example, radiation and chemotherapy are highly effective against Wilms' tumor, a childhood cancer that was once notoriously fatal. But Wilms' survivors frequently experience curved or stunted spines as a result of intensive radiation. Studies of Hodgkin's disease survivors indicate that standard doses of radiation to the head and neck can later produce thyroid dysfunction, dental complications, cataracts, and other long-term disabilities. In some cases, radiation and chemotherapy can even give rise to secondary tumors.

Although my own long-term effects were minimal — a

slight limp and chronic lymphedema — Lisa, my good friend and co-founder of Cancervive, wasn't so lucky. Aggressive radiation treatment for her ovarian cancer caused many serious complications. As you might expect, the issue of long-term effects is one of great concern to me — as it is with so many of the survivors I meet.

That is why I thought it important to include this chapter. I realize that a look at the long-term effects of treatment may come across to some readers as a kind of oncological house of horrors. The intention isn't to scare but rather to alert and inform survivors of some of the latent risks associated with current cancer therapy and to highlight a few treatment-related problems that, with proper follow-up, can be alleviated.

Unfortunately, some physicians tend to minimize these concerns; they view the lingering and late effects of cancer therapy as the inevitable price of being cured. Grace Christ, director of the department of social work at New York's Memorial Sloan-Kettering Cancer Center, explains why:

There is an ongoing dialogue within the medical community over the kinds of problems survivors have and how important they are. This is because physicians and survivors see the problem from two different perspectives. The physician's job is to treat the disease, with the goal of achieving remission. But the survivor has moved beyond that and is now faced with quality of life issues — issues some doctors may not relate to or understand.

Dr. Maurie Markman, a medical oncologist at Memorial Sloan-Kettering, believes that physicians *are* paying greater attention to patients' long-term difficulties. "Fortunately," he says, "we now have the luxury of talking about these problems."

People forget that oncology is a relatively new field of study. Many of the long-term effects that we see today are the result of the kinds of treatment used in the early days. Use of chemotherapy began in the fifties, but we didn't really achieve a full understanding of it until the seventies. Twenty years ago, no one could anticipate some of these later complications. We were just trying to cure as many people as we could, using the new and experimental treatments that were available to us at the time.

But many of those remissions came at a high price. As the complications of early cancer treatment became apparent, oncologists sought to minimize the effects by modifying existing therapies.

Dr. Frank L. Meyskens, Jr., director of the cancer center at the University of California–Irvine, stresses that oncologists are now carefully monitoring the dosage of anticancer drugs and radiation. They're also constantly on the lookout for newer, less toxic treatments. According to Dr. Meyskens, one of the more striking modifications in treatment involves the phasing out of the standard chemotherapy regimen known by the acronym MOPP (a combination of the chemotherapeutic drugs mechlorethamine [Mustargen], vincristine [Oncovin], procarbazine, and prednisone).

MOPP was the first really successful treatment against Hodgkin's disease, but we are replacing it now with ABVD [a combination of doxorubicin, bleomycin, vinblastine, and dacarbazine], which has a much lower rate of both short- and long-term effects, including less risk of second malignancies. The other modification we've made is in the treatment of lymphoma, both Hodgkin's and non-Hodgkin's. We used to treat these cases with both chemotherapy and extensive radiation. But we have significantly decreased the dose of radiation in many cases, and that has lowered the incidence of secondary problems in these patients.

Yet another example of treatment modification is in the use of tamoxifen, an anti-estrogen drug, in place of estrogen for breast cancer patients. "We used to use estrogen all the

time," says Dr. Meyskens, "which of course caused very difficult side effects for patients with postmenopausal breast cancer. Now we use the equally effective tamoxifen and the side
effects are one hundredth of what estrogen's used to be."

But not all treatment modifications are safer. The use of
new limb salvage techniques, organ-sparing procedures, and
bone marrow transplantations may actually increase the com-
plexity of cancer therapy, thereby increasing the potential for
late effects. Take the example of an adult patient with acute
leukemia who is in remission after standard treatment. Such
a patient might be an excellent candidate for bone marrow
transplantation, which frequently combines high-dose chemotherapy, immunosuppressive agents, and total body irradiation. Although this aggressive therapy provides the patient
with another chance at a cure, its potential for long-term consequences — such as rejection of bone marrow (graft-versus-
host disease) and infection — must be thoroughly considered.

In short, cancer therapy involves a delicate balance, and
both physician and patient must carefully weigh the risks
against the benefits of treatment. Says Dr. Markman:

> We now have a better understanding of some of the problems that
> resulted from earlier therapies. We've seen their long-term effects,
> and so we don't give those kinds of toxic doses anymore. But even
> though the goal is to reduce toxicity of treatment, it's critical that we
> don't reduce efficacy.

Surviving cancer is complicated by the fact that today's
treatment — although greatly improved over what was available twenty years ago — remains an inexact and evolving science. It is important for survivors to note that the long-term
effects of treatment vary widely and depend on the age of
the patient, the type and location of malignancy, the kind of
therapy used, and the intensity and duration of that therapy.
The more complex and intense a patient's treatment is, the

greater the chance of late complications. Whereas the effects of surgery are usually clear-cut and immediate, the cumulative effects of chemotherapy and radiation can take years to manifest themselves.

The Long-Term Effects of Chemotherapy

Chemotherapy, as most survivors know, involves the use of powerful and, in some cases, toxic chemicals to kill cancer cells. These drugs are often given in various potent combinations, euphemistically called "chemo cocktails." What makes many anticancer drugs so noxious is that they often don't distinguish between malignant cells and those that are healthy and normal.

Chemotherapy patients are told these drugs will alter their appearance, and perhaps their lives, in the short run. And although the immediate side effects are often unpleasant, they are measured against the treatment's ability to destroy cancer. Most patients agree that it's a fair trade, so they marshal their strength and dig in their heels. Once treatment is over, however, they expect these side effects to slowly ebb away. Most of them do, but occasionally survivors find they are left with physical reminders of the battle against cancer. Many of these lingering and late effects can be easily treated, but others pose more serious problems and may even be life-threatening.

Along with thousands of other cancer patients, Alice, twenty-six, received doxorubicin (Adriamycin) as part of an aggressive chemotherapy regimen for T-cell leukemia. Although she is delighted that the treatment seems to have cured her cancer, Alice says she wishes she had been more alert to the possible long-term side effects.

I was sixteen when I was diagnosed with leukemia. It took all of my strength to get through chemo. Once I was done, all I wanted was to put cancer behind me and get on with living. I felt that I had paid my dues.

I met Rick during my last year at college, and a year later we were married. My health was really never a topic of discussion. I was feeling fine, and I never thought much about cancer anymore.

Rick and I planned on having lots of children, so as soon as we settled down we decided to get started on a family. It didn't take long before I was pregnant. I was fine at first but after a few months, I noticed that I was having trouble getting through the day. I felt very weak and sort of sick and I didn't know why. My doctor thought it might have something to do with my hormones kicking up. But it didn't feel like that to me; this seemed different from anything I'd read about in the pregnancy books.

I was a little worried, but decided to ignore it. I kept thinking it would go away, that I was just having a hard pregnancy. But then one day while I was exercising, I became really short of breath and my heart started racing. I started wheezing, and I had trouble breathing.

I knew something was definitely wrong. Rick was home so he rushed me to my oncologist, who examined me and said that I was experiencing mild cardiac failure. He explained that one of the chemo drugs I'd received, Adriamycin, can be toxic to the heart during periods of extreme stress. I didn't consider exercising to be that stressful, but in my case it was.

I was confined to bed for the duration of my pregnancy and given special heart medication. My labor and delivery went okay, although the doctors monitored me very closely. I gave birth to a healthy baby boy.

When I think about what might have happened, I realize how lucky I was. I later found out that because my heart was so weak, I could have died during labor. My doctor said that this wouldn't have happened if I had been properly monitored from the start. Since then, I feel as if I've been given a second chance at staying healthy. I now get echocardiograms every year and I make a point to have regular checkups.

Like many survivors, Alice never fully understood how chemotherapy would continue to affect her life long after it had accomplished its job of knocking out cancer. Some anti-cancer drugs are more toxic than others and have a greater capacity for inflicting long-term damage on otherwise healthy organs. Both doxorubicin and daunorubicin (Cerubidine), two common antitumor antibiotics, can cause heart damage that in turn may lead to chronic congestive heart failure. The toxicity of these drugs depends on several factors, including the total dose given as well as the procedure used to administer the drug (that is, by bolus push instead of infusion).

Not every patient treated with these drugs develops later cardiac complications. In fact, patients with strong hearts are at very little risk for cardiotoxicity. Those most at risk include elderly patients (aged seventy or older), patients who have a history of hypertension or coronary heart disease, and those who have received previous irradiation to the chest or were given other cardiotoxic drugs. As Alice found out, cumulative congestive heart failure can take years to develop. Once it does, it may come on suddenly and is often triggered by extreme stress. Symptoms include shortness of breath, an inability to tolerate exercise, swelling of the legs and feet, a fast or irregular heartbeat, wheezing, and in some cases chest pain.

Physicians have known about the effects of these drugs for years but believe that their efficacy in fighting cancer is worth the risks. To alleviate potential problems, patients who are treated with cardiotoxic drugs are closely monitored throughout treatment. If and when heart damage does occur, many patients respond well to the use of heart medication such as digitalis. If you were treated with large doses of either Adriamycin or Cerubidine, don't wait for symptoms to tip you off. Be sure your follow-up exams include an electrocardiogram (EKG) and a serial echocardiogram, two noninvasive techniques used to assess and monitor heart activity.

These drugs aren't the only ones that cause later complications. Patients who receive bleomycin (Blenoxane) may be at risk for lung damage (pulmonary toxicity). Bleomycin can cause lung fibrosis, the formation of scar tissue in the lungs, which in turn can lead to a variety of respiratory problems.

The drug cisplatin, a relatively new chemotherapeutic agent, may produce kidney damage and hearing problems, including tinnitus (ringing in the ears) and hearing loss. The use of vincristine can result in nerve disorders such as extreme numbness in hands and feet as well as chronic jaw pain. Many of the chemotherapy drugs classified as alkylating agents (such as cyclophosphamide [Cytoxan] and mechlorethamine) are notable for their ability to damage genetic material.

None of this is to suggest that people treated with chemotherapy will necessarily develop late effects. On the contrary, many survivors bounce back from therapy and enjoy a long life, free of serious complications. But it is important to remember that any drug — even aspirin — has the capacity to cause harmful side effects. Good health requires a certain amount of vigilance, and this maxim is doubly true for survivors. Be alert to the fact that most chemotherapy drugs pose risks to long-term health — it is essential to monitor for them. When caught early, many of these problems can be successfully treated. Should any side effect from chemotherapy persist after treatment or new, unexplainable symptoms appear, notify your doctor immediately.

The Long-Term Effects of Radiation

Like chemotherapy, radiation therapy has its own set of acute side effects, most of which are confined to the part of the body being irradiated. Some of the more general short-term complications include skin burns, sores, fatigue, and hair loss. Many of these side effects subside shortly after treatment ends. As with chemotherapy, however, sometimes these complications are permanent, whereas others don't manifest themselves until much later.

When thirty-eight-year-old Jeremy first noticed symptoms of a glioblastoma (brain tumor) seven years ago, he was working as a certified public accountant for a large accounting firm. He underwent surgery to remove the tumor as well as six weeks of cranial radiation and chemotherapy. But several months into recovery, Jeremy realized that he was having treatment-related difficulties. He explains what happened:

I first noticed a problem one day when I sat down to write a few checks. Right away, I saw that I was having trouble doing simple calculations. I thought that maybe I was somehow off that day, and that I probably needed to take it easy. But a couple of months later, I was still having difficulties.

For someone trained as an accountant, the loss of such basic skills is upsetting, to put it mildly. My doctor suggested I see a psychologist, who then put me through a battery of tests. I learned a lot from those evaluation tests on how radiation had affected my thinking process. One test revealed that I had difficulty putting things in sequence, another pointed to memory problems. I called my neurologist and asked him what was going on. He informed me that it was probably caused by the radiation. He said I'd received the maximum dose, and that it may have caused some permanent damage.

Since then, as a result of the radiation, I've done some really whacked-out things. I remember going to a dinner party with some friends not too long ago. There was a bottle of champagne on the dinner table and next to it an empty champagne bucket. I stared at these two objects for a while, then picked up the bottle, opened it, and proceeded to empty it into the bucket. Everyone at the party watched in stunned silence. It took me a few minutes to realize what I had done, and then I was tremendously embarrassed. I still have no idea what got into my head. At the time it just seemed to make perfect sense.

I called my therapist the next day and she told me that somewhere in my brain I'd made a connection between the bottle and the ice bucket, but obviously it wasn't the right connection. She said that in my mind, emptying that champagne was the logical thing to do. It's just the way radiation has scrambled my thinking process. Fortunately, these accidents don't happen too often.

Thanks to impressive advances in technology, radiation therapy is now an effective weapon against certain types of formerly fatal brain tumors. But to achieve remission, high doses of radiation to the head are necessary. What is it about this kind of radiation treatment that causes these changes in the thinking process? Dr. Jordan Wilbur, head of pediatric oncology at the Children's Cancer Research Institute in San Francisco, explains:

In many ways the brain is like a computer. Each thought process involves millions of neural connections. If you received radiation to the head, some of the connections that deal with understanding certain concepts can get burned out. They simply don't connect anymore. In very young patients, those under age five or six, it's almost a hundred percent guaranteed that this will be the case. After this age, it depends on how much radiation is involved.

As with chemotherapy, radiation can batter normal body tissue while it goes about its mission of destroying cancer cells. Consequently, patients who receive irradiation to the head or the central nervous system frequently experience a minor decrease in I.Q. level and attention span and are at risk for other problems involving perception and motor skills. As Dr. Wilbur notes, young children are particularly vulnerable to later radiation-caused learning disabilities. Fortunately, many of these problems are remedial and can be corrected with early intervention.

The long-term effects of any radiation treatment depend on the location and the amount of the dose. Irradiation of the chest, for example, can lead to permanent scarring of the lungs. Children who receive high-dose radiation to the head and skeletal system may later experience problems in their growth and development. When the head is irradiated, the part of the brain that produces growth hormone, the pituitary gland, can be affected, resulting in a diminished growth rate for the young survivor. Radiotherapy to the spine, abdomen, or pelvis may also result in restricted growth. During follow-up, physicians monitor the growth pattern of such children and refer them to an endocrinologist if problems develop.

Intense radiotherapy can cause a multitude of other late complications, more than I can possibly list here. Again, it is your responsibility to learn about the potential problems that may result from your type of treatment and to discuss any late effect concerns with your oncologist.

Lymphedema

In some patients, radiation or surgery can injure or destroy lymph nodes and vessels under the arm or in the groin, resulting in the chronic swelling of a limb. This condition is called lymphedema and is the result of an accumulation of lymphatic fluid.

I first noticed the telltale signs of lymphedema three years after my treatment for rhabdomyosarcoma when my ankle and later my entire right leg began to swell. My doctor told me that high-dose radiation to my right thigh had resulted in permanent scarring of the lymphatic channels. Although the condition is painless, I've occasionally experienced serious infection in my right leg as a result of it.

Thanks to newer treatment techniques, the incidence of lymphedema is much lower today. Nevertheless, survivors who have had lymph nodes removed or have received radiation to an area containing lymph glands should watch for signs of lymphedema and take special precautions to guard against infection.

Diana's experience shows how this condition can crop up unexpectedly. Four years ago, the forty-eight-year-old airline executive was found to have a small malignant lump in her right breast. Diana chose to have a lumpectomy, followed by lymph node excision (the removal of lymph nodes surrounding the tumor). All nodes tested negative, but her oncologist

suggested a course of radiation as a protective measure.
Diana was relieved to know her cancer appeared to be under
control. But she wondered why no one warned her about
lymphedema.

My lumpectomy was a snap compared to the lymph node procedure. I woke up to find my right arm taped to my side with these
awful drainage tubes coming out of me. A few days later, after the
tubes and bandages were removed, the nurse told me that my arm
would be numb and tender for a while. She showed me how to do
several exercises to regain mobility in that arm. After that, I was
pretty much left to my own devices.

The radiation treatment was easy; except for the fatigue, I had
no real problems with it. But I was becoming more and more concerned about my arm. It continued to feel heavy and wooden. Then
one night I started getting dressed for a party. It was the first time
since my cancer treatment that I'd worn a long-sleeved dress. I
knew something was wrong when I tried to get my right arm
through the sleeve and it wouldn't fit. I took one look at my arm and
couldn't believe how swollen it was. My first thought was, Oh my
God. It's the cancer. It's back!

I immediately called my doctor at home. He tried to reassure me
by saying it was nothing serious, but I insisted he take a look at it. I
went to see him the next day, and he explained that I had a bad case
of lymphedema, that the swelling was due to a build-up of lymph
fluids. He suggested I control it with a tight compression sleeve and
that I be careful not to injure the arm in any way. He said that even
an insect bite to the area could cause serious infection.

I left his office feeling frustrated and helpless. I hated the idea of
having a chronically swollen arm. But since my doctor said there
was nothing I could do, I ignored it for a long time. It was much
easier for me to deny I had a problem. Also, I found it very hard to
accept that my little episode with breast cancer could result in my
arm being permanently disfigured.

But all that changed when my arm became seriously infected. I
had to be hospitalized, and to make a long story short, it scared me
into taking action. I realized that if I was going to have to live with
this for the rest of my life, I needed to find out all I could about it.

I attended a local mastectomy support group workshop. The
physical therapist conducting the workshop said there were ways of

treating lymphedema. She emphasized that it was very important not to ignore the condition. If the lymphedema was not managed, she said, the stagnant lymphatic fluid in my arm could eventually cause tissue to die.

Well, that was a rude awakening. My doctor had never told me that the condition could be so dangerous. I asked a lot of questions at that workshop and collected loads of printed material on lymphedema. Then I started researching the kind of treatments available. I found out about a company that sold a special compression pump that controlled the lymphedema by keeping the lymphatic fluid circulating. I tried it, and it worked like a charm. Since then, I've been using the pump three times a week and in between I wear a compression sleeve. It's not a cure, but it sure makes a difference.

Cancer patients frequently undergo removal of lymph nodes as part of their surgery. Follow-up radiation treatment can also damage lymphatic channels, resulting in the pooling of lymph fluid. When the circulation of this fluid slows down or stagnates, the affected limb becomes susceptible to infection. It is essential for survivors with lymphedema to do what they can to prevent even minor injury to the affected arm or leg.

Here are several precautionary steps you can take to avoid infection:

- *Protect the limb from any cuts or burns.* Protection requires special attention on your part, such as avoiding sunburn, using an electric razor instead of a blade for shaving, and wearing gloves during gardening or while doing the dishes. Insect or animal bites to the affected limb require prompt medical attention. Even something as innocuous as cutting your cuticles can result in infection.
- *Keep abrasions clean.* If the skin is cut or broken in any way, wash the area immediately with soap and water, apply antibacterial medication, and cover with a bandage.
- *Have doctors or nurses use only your unaffected arm for injections and blood pressure readings.* It's a good idea to carry with you a

special medical I.D. tag identifying your impaired limb (for example: LEFT ARM — LYMPHEDEMA) which will alert doctors and nurses to use the other limb for tests.

- *Watch out for pressure and fluid retention.* Keep clothing and jewelry loose to avoid pressure. Also, try to keep your weight down to lessen fluid retention.
- *Elevate the limb.* Rest the affected limb in an elevated position whenever possible to relieve swelling.
- *Exercise.* As important as it is to be careful of your impaired arm or leg, that doesn't mean you should baby it. Keep muscle tone up through regular exercise (including post-mastectomy exercises), but avoid overexerting the limb.
- *Watch for warning signals.* Contact your physician immediately if the affected area turns red, or becomes tender or painful.

As Diana discovered, there is no cure for lymphedema, but treatments to control the symptoms do exist. Survivors can benefit from a combination of two existing therapies: the use of a special pump followed by wearing an elastic compression garment (either stocking or sleeve). The pump applies gentle pressure to the affected area, forcing the lymphatic fluid to circulate back out of the limb and thereby decreasing the swelling. A support stocking or sleeve stimulates circulation and helps prevent fluid build-up. It works in much the same way support hose alleviate varicose veins.

When prescribed by a physician, compression pumps are covered by most insurance companies, but it is advisable to check with your company first. Shop around before buying a pump; ask that a sales representative visit you so that you can try the pump out before purchasing it. There are several types available, and one may work better for you than others. The National Lymphedema Network suggests the following retailers:

BIOCOMPRESSION SYSTEMS
736 Gotham Parkway
Carlstadt, NJ 07072
(800) 888-0908

HUNTLEIGH TECHNOLOGY, INC.
227 Route 33 East
Manalapan, NJ 07726
(800) 223-1218

JOBST INSTITUTE, INC.
653 Miami Street
Toledo, OH 43605
(800) 228-2736

LYMPHA PRESS
CAMP INTERNATIONAL
P.O. Box 89
Jackson, MI 49204
(800) 482-1088

WRIGHT LINEAR PUMP
185-A Robinson Road
Imperial, PA 15126
(800) 631-9535

Compression garments are not always covered by insurance. Contact your insurance company to find out what your coverage allows. Retailers for support sleeves and stockings include

BARTON CAREY
P.O. Box 421
Perrysburg, OH 43551
(800) 421-0444

JOBST INSTITUTE, INC.
653 Miami Street
Toledo, OH 43605
(800) 228-2736

JAMES KENDRICK CO.
6139 Germantown Avenue
Philadelphia, PA 19144
(800) 523-0178

SIGVARIS
P.O. Box 570
Branford, CT 06405
(800) 322-7744

WRIGHT LINEAR PUMP
185-A Robinson Road
Imperial, PA 15126
(800) 631-9535

JULIUS ZORN, INC.
P.O. Box 1088
Cuyahoga Falls, OH 44223
(800) 222-4997

For further information on the treatment of lymphedema, contact the National Lymphedema Network, a nonprofit resource center located at 2211 Post Street, Suite 404, San Francisco, Calif. 94115 (tel. 800-541-3259).

Chronic Fatigue

Fatigue is one of the hallmarks of cancer therapy. Patients expect radiation or chemotherapy to play havoc with their stamina. Fighting off a life-threatening disease is, after all, exhausting work. But once treatment ends, patients look forward to regaining all that hard-spent energy. Instead, months or even years later, they may find that they're still feeling run down, mustering all their reserves just to get through the day. Fatigue can be such a problem for some survivors that they find it hard to function at a normal level.

Jane Hawgood is a clinical social worker in radiation oncology at the University of California–San Francisco Medical Center. She is also an eleven-year survivor of breast cancer. Hawgood points out that the medical community is beginning to realize how debilitating chronic fatigue can be to recovered cancer patients.

Fatigue is a big problem for many cancer survivors. The medical community used to pass it off as a sign of depression; fatigue was seen strictly as an emotional problem. But we now realize that in many cases there are organic reasons for it. Doctors, nurses, and social workers are now discussing the problem of fatigue with patients and helping them find ways to cope with it.

Hawgood adds that there is a great deal of speculation about the causes of chronic fatigue in cancer survivors. Some believe it is brought about by the additional energy the body must expend on rebuilding injured cells. Others suspect that bone marrow suppression is responsible. After treatment, bone marrow recovery may be slow or incomplete, which in turn inhibits the production of infection-fighting white blood cells, oxygen-carrying red blood cells, and blood-clotting platelets. If your white blood count drops below normal, your body has to use more energy to fight infection and repair damaged cells. When your red blood count is too low, the body isn't getting all the oxygen it needs, which can result in anemia; in some instances it can become chronic. When your body has to make do with a reduced blood count, you can feel tired and run down.

Since the cancer experience is so emotionally draining and disruptive to a person's lifestyle, many physicians believe that a patient's lack of pep is caused by depression. To be sure, fatigue and listlessness are often the physical counterparts of grief or depression. If you think your lack of energy could have an emotional cause, you may want to get in touch with a support group or therapist. For some people, emotion-based fatigue is a temporary state; they learn to recognize why they are feeling low and find ways to pull themselves through the down times. For others, depression is a more deep-seated problem and therefore requires more serious attention.

"Many survivors find that coming to terms with fatigue means changing their lifestyle to fit their diminished energy level," explains Hawgood. "It may require accepting a new 'normal' level of activity." She adds that survivors who are struggling with chronic fatigue might want to consider the following suggestions:

- *Be in tune with your fatigue.* Try to understand when you are most likely to be affected by fatigue, then find ways of managing it. Give yourself permission to take naps. If naps don't suit you, experiment with other kinds of relaxation. Some survivors report that it helps to spend quiet time alone, meditating, reading, or just puttering around the house.
- *Try to organize your day so that you conserve as much energy as possible.* Determine what the most productive time of the day is for you and gauge yourself accordingly.
- *Don't try to do the impossible.* Some survivors attempt to maintain their old schedules and routines, then feel frustrated because they run out of steam before they've accomplished what they set out to do. Accept that your lack of energy is treatment-related and don't try to fight it. But don't let it defeat you either.
- *Maintain a healthy diet and exercise program.* If you aren't eat-

ing a well-balanced, nutritional diet, you're bound to feel run down sooner or later. Food is fuel. Make sure that the foods you eat provide you with the nourishment you need to maintain strength and energy. And don't overlook the importance of regular exercise as an antidote to low energy and an outlet for emotions. Exercise is an excellent way to build up strength and stamina after treatment.

The Risk of Secondary Tumors

Although the fear of recurrence lurks in the back of most survivors' minds, few give much thought to the chance of new or secondary tumors. However, this possibility should be of special concern to survivors of childhood cancer, who are surviving longer and are therefore at greater risk for developing late complications of their treatments.

I recently met a thirty-six-year-old survivor who knows all about those risks. Carla is a free-lance artist who, when she was one year old, was diagnosed with Wilms' tumor, a form of kidney cancer that primarily affects children. In the mid-fifties, treatment for Wilms' included surgery (in Carla's case, to remove her left kidney) followed by intensive radiation and chemotherapy. The treatment worked and her cancer was eradicated. But as Carla explains, she's been struggling with the consequences of that cure ever since.

My parents didn't tell me I had cancer until I was twelve. Even then, I never really got the details. Families deal with cancer in different ways. My family chose to deal with it by *not* dealing with it. By the time I was a teenager, I had become very angry and resentful that my family had handled my illness the way they did. For example, the radiation had affected growth on the left side of my torso. It also left me with a curved spine. A lot of things that could have been done in the way of reconstructive surgery were just never addressed.

I was thirty years old when, during a follow-up visit, I told my doctor about a hard lump I'd found in my right breast. I wasn't really worried about it though. I'd had many benign lumps removed over the years — from my breasts, my bladder, my back, you name it. So I thought this was probably just another noncancerous growth. Since I hadn't been warned about the risk of future secondary malignancies, I never considered cancer to be a possibility. I actually believed that since I'd already had the disease, I was safe.

When the doctor told me my breast lump was malignant, I refused to believe her. I went for a second opinion, and then a third. But there was no getting around it; I had cancer again. All the doctors said that the tumor "looked good" — I love that expression — and that other than a mastectomy, I wouldn't need any further treatment. Now that I think of it, I was still in denial right up to the time of the operation.

While I was recovering, my doctor explained how my early treatment for Wilms' may have precipitated this tumor — and that I could very well be at risk for further breast cancer. She gave me more information about late effects than I had ever received in my life. My doctor gave me the choice of whether to continue with intensive follow-ups and yearly mammograms or have the other breast removed as a precautionary measure. She wasn't pushy, but she strongly urged me to consider a second mastectomy.

My first reaction was "Forget it! I'd rather die than go through that." It was just too much too soon. I told my doctor I needed to think about it. And I did — for a year. I spent a lot of that year feeling sorry for myself. During this time I also had to deal with early menopause — another late effect surprise. With this and the earlier damage done by radiation — well, let's just say I was not a happy camper. I was carrying around a lot of anger and resentment and I didn't want to deal with the very real possibility of finding another malignant lump in my breast. It's a stupid attitude, I know. But that's how I felt.

It took me a long time to get beyond all that. I thought long and hard about it and finally realized that I was looking at a life-or-death decision. I went ahead with the operation and later had breast reconstruction surgery.

My doctor told me the tissue in that breast was precancerous, so I guess I made the right decision. But it wasn't easy. It was a major process for me to go from bitterness and complete denial to active decision making.

My attitude has totally changed since that second mastectomy. I'm much more assertive about my health. A close call with death makes you very aggressive.

The great irony of cancer treatment is that the methods used to cure patients can also lay the ground for future malignancies. Radiation, like certain chemotherapy drugs belonging to the alkylating group, can potentially cause a variety of secondary cancers, including leukemia, bone sarcomas, and thyroid cancer. Studies show that while the majority of survivors will remain free of their initial disease, their chances of contracting another cancer are about three times higher than that of the rest of the population.

This isn't to imply that cancer therapy is inadvisable. On the contrary, the efficacy of current forms of treatment cannot be underestimated. Without them there would undoubtedly be fewer treatment complications — and far fewer survivors. Half a million people are successfully treated for cancer each year, and of that number only a small percentage is at risk for treatment-induced malignancies.

Then again, not all relapses and secondary cancers are the result of treatment. Genetic tendencies and lifestyle habits, like smoking and high-fat diets, also play a role in whether a survivor will develop a secondary cancer. The study of long-term effects of treatment is so new that doctors still have difficulty identifying symptoms that are treatment-related and those that would have occurred regardless of therapy.

Dr. Jordan Wilbur adds:

The risk of secondary tumors is of concern, simply because a certain number of survivors contract them. Current statistics show that approximately five percent of survivors are likely to get treatment-induced cancers, or about one in twenty. However, for certain malignancies it's higher than that. The question is, do you want to be alive to have that worry? You have to put it in perspective.

Survivors need to remember that most cancers can be successfully treated if caught early. Annual checkups, preferably by a physician familiar with your cancer history, should be an important part of your life.

Although radiation and chemotherapy have proved to be successful in treating many forms of cancer, questions concerning their use remain. How much is too much? What is the danger point? How do we identify those survivors who are at greater risk? There are no easy answers. As Dr. Maurie Markman observes:

The issue is, how helpful is it to the survivor to worry about something that has an extremely limited chance of happening? How does one draw the line at what is in the patient's best interest? It is critical for survivors to know about the risks and to be vigilant, and it would be great if we could completely avoid the side effects. But don't forget that the goal of cancer treatment is to keep people alive.

When Anger Becomes a Long-Term Effect

The psychological turmoil created by cancer doesn't necessarily end with treatment. Rather, as a survivor, you are faced with new concerns, new challenges, and many more questions. What, if any, long-term effects will you encounter? If surgery has altered your appearance, how will you learn to accept your new body image? How can you best handle the anger and frustration over all the changes cancer has created in your life? The process of sorting through these issues can be a big job — one that many survivors approach with a great deal of bitterness. As Carla says:

All cancer patients realize that some kind of price must be paid for exacting a cure. I don't think anyone honestly expects to emerge from the experience unscathed. But most of us thought that the worst was over once treatment ended. For many of us it isn't, and yet we're supposed to grin and bear it.

You may feel embarrassed or guilty about the anger you are feeling. You might even think you aren't entitled to these emotions. I know I felt that way after I developed lymphedema. Once I was free of cancer, everyone expected me to be beyond any emotional pain or resentment over treatment side effects. But that was much easier said than done.

Jeremy, the former accountant introduced earlier in this chapter, also continues to wrestle with the emotional and physical aftermath of cancer therapy. Although his brain tumor has been in remission for six years, his anger has been harder to contain.

The most difficult part of my recovery was adjusting to the effects of treatment. Since my cancer I've become totally dependent on my family for everything. I am unable to return to my former line of work. My depth perception and motor skills have been affected to the point where I can no longer drive a car. My life is so different now, and some days that's very hard for me to accept.

I'm still angry that my doctors never gave me the full picture on how treatment might affect me. I'm sure that I would have still gone through with it and taken my chances, but at least I would have felt that it was a shared decision. When you haven't been warned, and then all of a sudden these things come out of left field and turn your life upside down, it's terribly discouraging. Once you stop feeling sorry for yourself, you get depressed and angry. And sometimes you stay that way.

Therapy has helped me learn how to find an outlet for my anger. Also, I'm taking special education classes every day for some of the problems treatment caused, and that's helped me refocus my thoughts. I enjoy swimming, so when I'm feeling upset, I'll go for a long swim and that relieves some of the stress. Other times, I'll just shut myself up in a room and yell and scream for a few minutes. That works the best.

Some illnesses are fairly easy to put behind us, but cancer isn't one of them. Once you've been diagnosed, cancer becomes a part of your identity. If the disease or its treatment has created physical disabilities or altered your body image, you will undoubtedly react with anger. And as Carla, Jeremy, and I discovered, that anger can be very hard to shake.

I now know that my anger had its roots in how the disease changed the view I had of myself. Cancer had a profound influence on my life, and it took a long time for me to adjust to and accept those changes. I needed to find ways of coming to terms with what I had lost and acknowledge that the loss was beyond my control. I couldn't go back in time to retrieve it. Instead I had to find a way to accept what had happened, renew myself, and get on with the job of living.

The danger comes, I realized, when survivors allow themselves to get mired in anger. If you don't find a way of dealing with it, anger can have a very corrosive effect on your life. Resentment can be dangerous in other ways as well simply because it is one of those emotions that almost always seeks out a target — doctors, family, friends, even ourselves. Most of us would admit that it's hard to feel good about ourselves when we have alienated those around us. The process of taming that great ogre within takes time and a certain amount of soul-searching.

FINDING WAYS TO TAKE CHARGE OF ANGER

Barbara J. Carter is a mental health registered nurse and research scientist who has studied the issues of cancer survivorship extensively. Anger, she stresses, is healthy, provided you use it productively:

Anger is one of those emotions that acts like a signpost; it signifies that something important has happened to us, and it should be heeded. It tells us that we have experienced a violation or a betrayal or a need that hasn't been met. Unfortunately, our culture has influenced most of us to think that anger is a bad emotion, and certainly not one we should express. But that kind of thinking can lead to lots of trouble later on. The best way to deal with anger is to find a constructive outlet for it. Get it to work for you, not against you.

I have found, as have many Cancervive members, that the best way to come to grips with anger — or any strong emotion for that matter — is to face it head on. This may be frightening to you, even unacceptable. As Carter notes, many of us learn from an early age to keep a lid on our emotions — especially volatile ones like anger. Others view the expression of anger as a sign of weakness, or as a violation of good manners. But bottled-up anger behaves a lot like the contents of a pressure cooker. Unless you find a way to let off steam, your anger will eventually cause you to explode, and that explosion is bound to injure a lot of innocent bystanders.

For many people, anger most often takes the form of blame or self-reproach. Some of the angriest survivors are those who, like Carla and Jeremy, were never told that they might have problems as a result of treatment. These survivors frequently end up blaming themselves for what they perceive to be their own inherent shortcomings.

Jeremy, for instance, says that because no one informed him that his radiation therapy might lead to short-term memory loss, his recovery was doubly frustrating.

It took me months to figure out that my memory problems were due to treatment. It's a very strange sensation, feeling like you've lost some of your brain power. Sometimes I feel a bit senile, the way I forget things all the time. I used to think it was just me, and I was real hard on myself. But then I found out through a support group that many other survivors who have received radiation to the head suffered from similar problems. That made me feel a hell of a lot better.

Dr. Patricia Ganz, director of the University of California–Los Angeles Cancer Rehabilitation Project, observes:

Survivors need to know that some of the difficulties they are experiencing may be related to their treatment. Studies show that many survivors of childhood malignancies were never even told they were treated for cancer. They had no way of knowing later on why they were having learning difficulties or problems with physical growth. It can help allay a lot of anxiety for these survivors to know that there are legitimate medical reasons for their problems.

Then again, some survivors say, "I was never told about these things," when in fact they *are* told what to expect before treatment begins, but they just don't hear it. They are so focused on getting through treatment that they block it out. Then when these problems surface later on, there is an initial sense of shock, followed by strong feelings of anger and resentment.

Even those patients who do understand and accept the potential risks involved may become upset and depressed when complications occur. They find themselves grappling with the resentment they feel toward their physicians, toward life, even toward their own bodies for betraying them. Says Grace Christ:

I think some of the frustration survivors feel is due in part to the difficulty they have getting doctors to pay attention to their post-treatment concerns. It helps to understand that some oncologists find it hard to address the topic of late effects. Their daily preoccupation revolves around trying to save lives. Many also have difficulty accepting that certain treatments do cause later problems. That's why it's so important for survivors to heighten the awareness of the medical community by reporting any late effects to their physicians.

Some recovered patients find the only way they can resolve their emotional turmoil is by communicating how they feel to their physicians. I am not suggesting that you and your doctor get into a screaming match. Instead, find time when you can both sit down and calmly discuss the repercussions of your treatment. Such an exchange may put to rest some of your resentment and anger and help speed your emotional recovery.

Years ago, Lisa and I decided to pay a visit to the radiation therapist who had treated us at Stanford University Medical Center. We went looking for answers to the many questions we had about the late effects of radiotherapy. We also wanted to vent our frustration over how treatment complications were affecting our lives. As you might imagine, it was a very emotional meeting — and, to our surprise, very cathartic.

Of course, if you choose to have this kind of discussion with your doctor, bear in mind that it may not go the way you planned. Some doctors simply aren't comfortable discussing patients' emotional problems. Also, be aware that you and your doctor are likely to have different perceptions of your cancer experience, so don't expect to see eye to eye on everything. Try to gauge how open your physician is to what you have to say. If your doctor is not responsive to your concerns, don't hesitate to find one who is.

It may also help if both you and your doctor share your experience with the entire medical team. This kind of informal "conference" will also give you a chance to further enlighten the medical community to the common and recurring biomedical issues associated with surviving cancer. By sharing your experience you'll find that the medical team will be more open and available to help with any future problems you have with late effects.

Barbara Carter notes that anger is energy, and it should be used constructively. Try to funnel your anger into a productive way of taking care of your needs. That's what Carla did:

I don't know if I'll ever stop feeling some bitterness over what happened to me, but at least I've found a way to handle it. I've been going to support group meetings for the past year, and that's been a big help. When I'm with the group I can express all that pain and frustration with people who understand. I've learned how to use visualization techniques, positive thinking, all that stuff. I've also pulled my head out of the sand. Now I make sure that I'm as informed and as knowledgeable as possible whenever I'm faced with an important decision. I've really taken it upon myself to be my own advocate — and that's made me feel much more confident about myself.

Living with Compromise

Recovery from cancer often involves adjusting to the loss of a body part. Amputation is of course a terrible blow to one's self-image. Losing a breast, a limb, a larynx is traumatic — an attack on your physical integrity. Part of you has been altered, and as a result you may feel diminished, no longer the same person. Other disabilities, such as loss of I.Q. points or infertility, while less obvious, are no less injurious to your self-esteem.

Says Barbara Carter, "Because of permanent physical alterations, some survivors will continue to live out their cancer experience for the rest of their lives. Humpty Dumpty can never be the same again."

She is referring to the "Humpty Dumpty syndrome," an apt description of the post-treatment cancer patient. The term was coined by Dr. Fitzhugh Mullan, co-founder of the National Coalition for Cancer Survivorship. Dr. Mullan, himself a survivor, uses this expression to describe how a recovering patient strives to regain a sense of normality after cancer, to piece life back together again. Eventually, the survivor learns to accept that the pieces may not fit the way they did before.

How do you come to terms with this newly reconstructed view of yourself? Many survivors find that physical or occupational therapy gives them the assistance they need to readapt comfortably. Sometimes physical rehabilitation, such as breast reconstruction, can be a positive step toward accepting a new body image. Of course, restorative rehabilitation is no magic act. It isn't going to improve every aspect of your life automatically. But it may very well improve your self-image, and that can make a big difference in how you approach life. Carter adds:

Coming to terms with a new self-image is an experience that is different for every individual. Each of us has very distinct notions concerning our body image, that is, who we are physically. When your body undergoes a dramatic change, you need to completely revamp your self-image — and that isn't easy. First you need to work through the grieving process and accept the loss of your former self. Once you've allowed that to happen, you can begin to reconstitute a new view of yourself through the cancer experience.

A part of that process involves the reactions and support of other people, especially family and friends. Their response will help shape your new outlook. By coming to terms with the feelings of friends and loved ones and infusing them with your own, you can slowly start to reassemble a new self-image.

Roaring down the road of recovery, years after their cancer experience, most survivors still find themselves glancing in the rearview mirror, checking out where they've been and who they've become. This process of integrating a new body image — that is, coming to terms with the physical aspects of the cancer experience — can take a long time, sometimes a lifetime. If that's happening to you, consider it normal; acceptance comes in small increments. Jane Hawgood found this to be true for herself:

You may need lots of time to mourn the physical loss — whether it's your prostate, your breast, your hair, or your former stamina. You have to experience the shock and the grief, the sadness and the anger, before you can get to the point where you can then say, "Okay. This is how it is. Now let's get on with life." With some losses, like mastectomies, it can take even longer to get to that point. I know that a lot of women say — as I did — "Hey, I'm okay. It really doesn't bother me." But it does. We put on a brave face because we feel a lot of pressure to be normal again. It can be especially hard to come to terms with your loss if the people around you are denying it. It's up to you to push beyond that denial and find ways of re-affirming your own positive perceptions of who you are.

Three years after the discovery of her lymphedema, Diana has learned how to adjust to what she calls her "oversized arm."

It used to be painful for me to even look at my right arm. Some-times it would get so swollen it looked deformed. I would try to hide it under loose clothing or just pretend that it didn't exist. Deep down, I knew I was rejecting this part of my body because it was cosmetically unappealing.

It took a serious infection for me to wake up to the fact that by ignoring my lymphedema I was jeopardizing my life. A small scratch to my right arm developed into a serious bacterial infection known as cellulitis. Fortunately it responded to antibiotics, but it really shook me up. I knew then that I had to take control of the situation. That's when I started using an extremity pump regularly and wear-ing a compression sleeve daily. It made such a difference; my arm became considerably thinner and felt less wooden and cumbersome.

That in turn helped me feel better about myself. I wasn't so self-conscious anymore, and I didn't feel so helpless. I think that by taking responsibility for my lymphedema I also took ownership of it.

Carla says that by accepting the physical changes brought about by cancer, she has become a much stronger person:

Since my double mastectomy, I've realized how becoming a cancer survivor put me in a completely new category of human beings. All of the coping I've done has really steeled me, made me a lot tougher. I'm more in control of my life now than I have ever been. I'll admit, sometimes depression will come creeping up on me. That's when I'll hightail it to a support group meeting. If that's not possible, I'll call up Mimi, a friend I met through the group. Mimi has gone through three bouts of cancer since she was a child, and like me, she's had a double mastectomy. We'll spend the first twenty minutes bitching and moaning about life, but that doesn't last. Mimi's got a great sense of humor and before long she'll have me in stitches. Norman Cousins was right, laughter is therapeutic. Somehow it gives me the emotional space I need to focus on the big picture.

The Importance of Follow-up

No one is immune to illness; everyone is at some risk of getting cancer. But as a survivor, you live with heightened risks. That is why comprehensive follow-up exams are so important. But Dr. Meyskens has observed that more than a few survivors prefer to ignore follow-ups:

Some recovered patients don't want to be reminded of their disease and so they avoid regular checkups. Those are the people who will be more at risk for later problems. Concerned survivors, on the other hand, are going to be more active in their health care and will have a much better chance of catching problems early.

Granted, one of the last things any of us wants to do is spend more time in a hospital or doctor's office. Your foot-dragging over follow-ups may be compounded by the anxiety you feel over returning to the hospital — the place you associate most with cancer. Or you could be worried about what may show up on tests. Even though these emotions are to be expected, they aren't always easy to overcome. If returning to "the scene of the crime" gives you the creeps, talk it over with a member of your health care team or with another survivor.

It might help if you remind yourself that medical checkups are preventative medicine — the best possible insurance for your new-found health. They also provide you with an opportunity to touch base with your physician, ask questions, and catch up on any late-breaking news regarding your type

of cancer. Remember that even though checkup exams are
hard on your nerves, they can also be an important source of
reassurance, with negative test results providing you with a
clean bill of health.

But that's not all. Not only are your checkups valuable for
safeguarding your health, but they also provide the medical
community with documentation of possible long-term effects.
Your feedback during checkups will facilitate further modification of treatment for future patients.

The responsibility for follow-up care doesn't lie solely with
survivors however; the medical community must also take a
more active role in attending to the long-term needs of recovered cancer patients. Susan Leigh is a registered nurse who
serves as a consultant with the National Coalition for Cancer
Survivorship. She believes the medical community has been
slow to address the long-term health concerns of survivors:

Very few hospitals are offering any real rehabilitation programs for
cancer patients. And yet cardiac patients, who have a much higher
chance of dying from their disease than do cancer patients, have all
kinds of comprehensive rehabilitation programs in place.

I think the medical community is obligated to establish follow-up
clinics that are appropriate to the needs of all long-term survivors.
We're losing people through the current system because many survivors just aren't coming back for their yearly checkups, and it's so
important that they do. And I'm not talking about just doing lump
and bump checks once a year. Survivors should have physical exams
that are tailored to their specific needs, and right now that's not
being done. Instead, most survivors are having to formulate their
own health maintenance programs.

Bear in mind that even though your doctor has declared
you disease-free, that doesn't mean you can simply drop out
of the health care system. Even years after recovery, you
should still consider yourself a key member of your treatment team. It's important that you keep in touch and stay informed. Dr. Julie Katz, director of the long-term effects clinic

at Children's Medical Center of Dallas, recommends the medical follow-up guidelines listed in the table on pages 217–219. Also, if you haven't already done so, find ways of making your life healthier, whether that means changing your diet or looking into stress-reduction techniques. Even the smallest changes can have far-reaching effects. It might help if you think of your body as a finely tuned machine. Doctors can perform maintenance and overhauls, but it's your job to look after the daily upkeep.

Late Effects Clinics

A few hospitals and medical centers around the country have established late effects clinics within their oncology departments. That these centers exist is an auspicious indication that the medical community is beginning to accommodate the need for long-term follow-up of cancer survivors. Because most survivorship research has focused on the pediatric cancer population, however, these clinics are primarily geared toward young survivors. Recovered patients of any age may nevertheless consult with the late effects specialists who are affiliated with these clinics.

LONG-TERM FOLLOW-UP CLINIC
Children's Hospital of Los Angeles
4650 Sunset Boulevard
Los Angeles, CA 90027
(213) 660-2450

LONG TERM FOLLOW-UP CLINIC
Children's Hospital of Philadelphia
34th Street and Civic Center Boulevard
Philadelphia, PA 19104
(215) 590-1000

LONG-TERM FOLLOW-UP CLINIC
Children's Medical Center of Dallas
1935 Motor Street
Dallas, TX 75235
(214) 920-2382

POST-TREATMENT RESOURCE PROGRAM
Memorial Sloan-Kettering Cancer Center
410 East 62nd Street
New York, NY 10021
(212) 639-3292

PEDIATRIC LONG TERM FOLLOW-UP CLINIC
Roswell Park Cancer Center
Carlton and Elm Streets
Buffalo, NY 14263
(716) 845-4447

AFTER COMPLETION OF THERAPY CLINIC
St. Jude Children's Research Hospital
332 North Lauderdale Drive
Memphis, TN 38101
(901) 522-0561

MEDICAL FOLLOW-UP GUIDELINES FOR LONG-TERM EFFECTS

Type of Treatment	Organs Affected	Screening Tests	Other Suggestions
		SURGERY	
Nephrectomy	Kidney	Chemistry profile Urinalysis Blood pressure checks	Refrain from excessive use of salt Maintain a healthy weight Exercise moderately Avoid contact sports
Splenectomy	Spleen	Blood count	May be placed on prophylactic antibiotics Avoid contagious diseases See your doctor for any fever over 101.5° F.
		RADIATION	
Abdomen	Kidney Liver Bladder	Chemistry profile Urinalysis Urine cytology every 3–5 years beginning 10 years after therapy ends Blood pressure checks	Avoid drinking alcohol Refrain from using salt Maintain a healthy weight Exercise moderately
Chest	Lungs Breast	Pulmonary function tests if short of breath Annual breast exam by a doctor Mammogram periodically after age 25	Do not smoke Self breast exam monthly Eat a low-fat diet
Head/neck	Eyes Teeth Thyroid	Eye exam yearly Dental exam every 6 months Palpation of thyroid yearly by a doctor Thyroid function tests as clinically indicated	Good oral hygiene
Groin/lower abdomen	Testes Ovaries	Sperm count	Do not delay childbearing if having regular periods

Type of Treatment	Organs Affected	Screening Tests	Other Suggestions
		CHEMOTHERAPY	
Adriamycin	Heart	EKG	Consult a doctor before beginning an exercise program or becoming pregnant
ARA-C	Liver (rare)	Chemistry profile	Avoid drinking alcohol
BCNU	Sex organs	Sperm count	Do not delay childbearing if having regular periods
Cis-platin	Kidneys Bladder Sex organs	Chemistry profile Urinalysis Urine cytology every 3–5 years beginning 10 years after therapy ends Blood pressure checks Sperm count	Avoid drinking alcohol Do not delay childbearing if having regular periods Refrain from using salt Maintain a healthy weight Exercise moderately
Cytoxan	Kidneys Bladder Sex organs	Chemistry profile Urinalysis Urine cytology every 3–5 years beginning 10 years after therapy ends Blood pressure checks Sperm count	Avoid drinking alcohol Do not delay childbearing if having regular periods Refrain from using salt Maintain a healthy weight Exercise moderately
Daunorubicin	Heart	EKG	Consult a doctor before beginning an exercise program or becoming pregnant
DTIC	Liver	Chemistry profile	Limit drinking alcoholic beverages
Ifosfamide	Kidney Bladder	Chemistry profile Urinalysis Urine cytology every 3–5 years beginning 10 years after therapy ends Blood pressure checks	Refrain from using excessive salt Maintain a healthy weight Exercise moderately
L-Asparaginase	Liver (rare) Pancreas (rare)	Chemistry profile	Limit drinking alcoholic beverages

Type of Treatment	Organs Affected	Screening Tests	Other Suggestions
		CHEMOTHERAPY (continued)	
Leukeran	Sex organs	Sperm count	Do not delay childbearing if having regular periods
Methotrexate	Liver	Chemistry profile	Limit drinking alcoholic beverages
Mustargen	Sex organs	Sperm count	Do not delay childbearing if having regular periods
Procarbazine	Sex organs Liver Kidney	Sperm count Chemistry profile Urinalysis	Do not delay childbearing if having regular periods Limit drinking alcohol Refrain from using excessive salt Maintain a healthy weight
6-Thioguanine (6-TG)	Liver	Chemistry profile	Limit drinking alcoholic beverages
Vincristine	Liver	Chemistry profile	Limit drinking alcoholic beverages
Blood transfusions	Liver Immune system	Chemistry profile HIV test may be indicated if transfused before 1985 Risk of non-A non-B hepatitis	Avoid drinking alcohol Practice safe sex

9

Longing for Life:
Cancer Treatment and Infertility

OF ALL the necessary losses caused by cancer treatment, perhaps none is as poignant as the loss of fertility. Surgery,
chemotherapy, radiation, and hormone therapy can all play
havoc with a cancer patient's reproductive system. Fortunately,
for many people this effect is temporary. But some aren't so
lucky; in their battle to sustain life, the potential for future
life is lost.

For many young survivors like myself, the double blow of
cancer and infertility can be overwhelming, or at the very
least color one's outlook on dating and marriage. Some Cancervive members have even told me that infertility presented
a much larger crisis in their lives than cancer ever did. Ms.
Michael Hubner, an oncology social worker at Boston's Beth
Israel Hospital, explains why:

For some survivors, coming to terms with infertility means coming
to terms with their cancer experience all over again and reliving

that deep sense of loss and grief. It reminds them of their vulnerability and may revive long dormant and unresolved emotions.

This is especially true of survivors of childhood cancer, many of whom were never told that treatment would make them sterile. They had to find out about their infertility on their own, years after they were treated, and it caused a real crisis in their lives. Even though they are considered cured, the majority of these survivors can't help but feel that, because of the infertility issue, cancer is continuing to influence their lives.

Of course, not every survivor faces the prospect of permanent sterility. And for some, the inability to have children is not a major concern. How a survivor will react to news of iatrogenic, or treatment-caused, infertility largely depends on the age as well as the life plan of that person. But if you're reading this chapter, chances are treatment-induced infertility is a concern in your life, and quite possibly a major one.

It certainly was for Kevin and Linda, two Cancervive members who triumphed over cancer only to learn that their victory had exacted the bitter compromise of infertility. Through their stories, we will examine the causes of both male and female infertility, as well as options for the infertile survivor.

Male Infertility: Kevin's Story

The ability to conceive children is a feat most couples take for granted. When that ability is forfeited, it can cause tremendous stress in a marriage, especially when it comes on the heels of a life-threatening crisis like cancer.

It's a problem Kevin knows all too well. When he was diagnosed with testicular cancer ten years ago, Kevin, now thirty-eight, never gave much thought to how it might affect the rest of his life. Even when he was told that treatment could leave him sterile, Kevin and his wife weren't overly concerned. Like any couple facing a cancer diagnosis, they concentrated all their attention on the immediate crisis looming before them.

Cindy and I had been married only a year, and kids weren't really part of our plan then. At the time, neither of us thought that something like my being sterile could make that much of a difference, as long as we had each other. But a few years later, as our marriage began to unravel, I realized how shortsighted we'd been.

My cancer was a seminoma, a form of testicular cancer. I had an undescended testicle, which had never been corrected. The surgeon removed it along with some lymph nodes and then, once that had healed, I was given radiation treatments. I never feared death; our only real concern was making sure I got through treatment okay. I'm just lucky I had Cindy to be there for me.

Before the operation my doctor suggested that I try sperm-banking. I'm glad I followed up on his suggestion. When I think about it now, that was really such a fateful decision, and yet I almost blew it off. Both Cindy and I were struggling to make ends meet, and at the time the issue of kids was easier left undiscussed.

At the sperm bank I was tested and they told me that my sperm sample was low. I asked my doctor about it, and he said to go ahead and make a deposit anyway. So I did, even though I didn't see much point in it.

My doctor was right about one thing: treatment left me sterile. At first, neither Cindy nor I really talked about it. Instead, once I'd bounced back, we both threw ourselves into work. I think the issue was still too sensitive for us to want to discuss it. But as time went on, I could feel the bitterness building up between us. Cindy was angry at me for depriving her of the chance to have kids, and I was angry at my parents. I felt that their neglect had caused the cancer. I also blamed the doctors, even though I knew it was sort of an irrational thing to do. It's just that cancer treatment left me feeling so inferior, so insecure about my masculinity. I took a lot of my anger out on my wife, and that just made things worse.

During one of my checkups, my doctor suggested we try having a baby through artificial insemination, using the sperm sample I'd banked. Cindy went through all the tests and we both spent a lot of time at the infertility clinic, trying to make a go of it. But it didn't seem to be working; my sperm sample wasn't up to speed. I guess I'd known that going in, but I figured you've got to try anyway, right?

The stress of it really started getting to us, though. We talked about adopting a baby, but the adoption process intimidated me, and Cindy wasn't wild about it either. We both felt so frustrated. It was like the whole infertility thing was strangling our marriage. We were close to calling it quits, but Cindy said she wanted to see another infertility specialist and give it one more try.

This time, Cindy underwent *in vitro* fertilization, using my sperm sample. Needless to say, when my wife saw the doctor for follow-up, we were expecting to hear bad news. So when Cindy came home and told me that she was pregnant, I could hardly believe it. I believe it now, though, and the proof is running around our house in the form of our five-year-old daughter, Annie.

CANCER TREATMENT AND MALE INFERTILITY

When it comes to cancer, Kevin is the first to admit that he's one of the lucky ones. When he was diagnosed, oncologists were just beginning to understand how to treat testicular cancer successfully. At the time, survival was by no means a sure thing. Today, however, the survival rate for this form of malignancy is between 70 and 80 percent.

Unfortunately, the likelihood that treatment will result in sterility is also high. Certain forms of radical surgery to a man's pelvic or abdominal area can damage pelvic nerves and lymphatics, which may cause problems with fertility and sexual functioning. During Kevin's surgery for testicular cancer his doctors removed several lymph nodes from the surrounding pelvic area so that they could determine if his cancer had spread. This procedure, called retroperitoneal lymph node dissection, can disrupt sensitive nerve connections that may in turn lead to a reduced ability to ejaculate. Surgery for colon cancer (colostomy), prostate cancer (prostatectomy), and bladder cancer (radical cystectomy) can also cause nerve damage to the penis, resulting in impaired fertility or altered sexual functioning.

The extent to which radiotherapy will affect a man's fertility depends primarily on the location of treatment and the total radiation dose. In many cases, men who receive radiation to the abdominal or pelvic area will experience either partial or full recovery of sperm production. But for some men, especially those who receive full-dose radiation to the gonads, infertility is often permanent.

In both males and females, sterility may occur if radiation treatment causes permanent damage to the pituitary gland. Located at the base of the brain, the pituitary gland is often referred to as the "master gland" because it directs the body's hormonal output, including those hormones that stimulate sperm production (in males) and egg maturation (in females). As a result, sufficient irradiation to a patient's head may cause the pituitary gland to function abnormally, which in turn will throw hormonal production out of whack.

Because of the toxic nature of some anticancer drugs, chemotherapy can interfere with both male fertility and sexual functioning, although in most instances these problems will disappear soon after treatment. But the effect of chemotherapy is not uniform. Its effect on fertility depends on the class and dose of the drugs as well as the age of the patient. Survivors who received chemotherapy for bone sarcomas, Hodgkin's disease, non-Hodgkin's lymphoma, and leukemia are most at risk for permanent damage to their reproductive organs. A class of chemotherapy drugs known as alkylating agents appears to be the main culprit in chemo-related sterility. Among these, the commonly used drug cyclophosphamide (Cytoxan) is perhaps the most notorious. Other drugs known to suppress fertility are chlorambucil (Leukeran), bulsulfan (Myleran), and vinblastine (Velban).

Male survivors who suspect that treatment has caused problems with their fertility can ask their doctors to provide them with two simple tests: a semen analysis and a blood test. Through semen analysis, the physician will be able to determine sperm count and motility as well as other factors that can interfere with fertility. A blood hormone test will also detect the levels of essential male hormones in the body, including testosterone, follicle-stimulating hormone (FSH), and luteinizing hormone (LH). Every man needs sufficient levels of all three hormones for sperm production to take place.

A reminder: although chemotherapy or radiation may have diminished or interrupted your sperm count or motility, this does not necessarily mean that you are unable to father children. In other words, don't rely on the effects of treatment as a method of birth control, especially if you are currently undergoing radiation or chemotherapy. If you have recently finished chemotherapy, your doctor may advise you or your partner to continue using some form of contraception since the effects of treatment on the reproductive system may linger for a year or more.

SEMEN CRYOPRESERVATION
AND SPERM BANKING

The easiest way for men to preserve their fertility prior to radiation or chemotherapy is to store samples of their semen at a sperm bank. This method of freezing and storing sperm is called semen cryopreservation, and an increasing number of male patients are electing to use this procedure as a way of preserving fertility. The man's sperm can then be used to fertilize a woman's egg through cervical insemination, gamete intra-Fallopian transfer, or *in vitro* fertilization (described later in this chapter).

Semen cryopreservation is particularly important to the male survivor whose initial cancer treatment was limited to surgery, but who may require additional treatment with chemotherapy or radiation in the future. For some male survivors, however, sperm banking is not always an option. A man may arrange to bank sperm before treatment begins, only to learn that cancer has already caused a reduction in either the concentration

or the motility of sperm. This little-understood phenomenon
is called subfertility. Doctors speculate that it is one of the
early effects cancer has on the body, a consequence of the disease's ability to depress levels of the hormones needed for
proper functioning of the reproductive system.

Your oncologist or primary-care physician can arrange to
have you tested to determine if your sperm production is
within the range acceptable for semen cryopreservation. If
tests reveal that you are subfertile, you should still consider
sperm banking as an option before you begin radiation or
chemotherapy. Like Kevin, many men have fathered children from subfertile sperm samples.

Survivors interested in obtaining more information about
sperm banks and their locations in North America should
contact the American Association of Tissue Banks, 1350 Bev-
erly Road, Suite 220-A, McLean, Va. 22101, (703) 827-9582.
The association also publishes a thirty-two-page booklet that
covers standards for cryobanking of sperm.

Female Infertility: Linda's Story

It is one thing to be warned at the time of diagnosis that cancer treatment will impair your fertility and quite another to
find out years later — on your own. When twenty-two-year-
old Linda came to her first Cancervive meeting more than a
year ago, the issue of infertility was foremost in her mind.
Like most teenagers, Linda wasn't sure what she wanted to be
when she grew up. But she was sure of one thing: she wanted
children. An only child, Linda promised herself that she
would compensate for her lack of siblings by one day having
a large family of her own.

When Linda was diagnosed with Hodgkin's disease at sixteen, she had no idea that treatment might affect her ability

to fulfill that dream. Her parents were informed, but they held back on telling their daughter. Instead they decided to wait until after her recovery to break the news. But that time never came, and Linda was left to figure it out for herself.

I was treated with the MOPP [Mustargen, Oncovin, procarbazine, and prednisone] regimen of chemotherapy along with radiation. I bounced back pretty fast from it all. The only thing was that my periods stopped shortly after my last treatment. I didn't think it was any big deal since my doctor had warned me that chemotherapy would probably cause some irregularity. I actually enjoyed having a break from my monthly periods. But no one said it would be a permanent thing. More than a year later, I still wasn't menstruating, so I went to see a gynecologist. He was the first person to lay it on the line: my treatment had resulted in complete ovarian dysfunction and it was unlikely I'd ever have kids.

At first I didn't believe him. Neither my oncologist nor my parents had ever told me that this would happen, so why should I believe a gynecologist? But as I drove home, everything he said began to sink in. By the time I got home, I was in a rage. That night I really ripped into my parents, yelling and screaming and accusing them. My mom just sat there crying. My dad tried to explain, saying that they had wanted to tell me, but they also wanted to spare me any more pain. The way I see it, holding back that kind of information just made it worse.

I haven't had an easy time adjusting to the loss. It hurts so much when I think about it. I've lost a part of me, a part of my future, and now I've got to learn to make do. Sometimes I think I would have rather given up an arm or a leg in exchange for healthy ovaries. That's how strongly I feel about it.

My biggest problem now is dating. It's a major hassle trying to tell a guy about all these things going on with me. If I ever do become serious about someone, I worry about how it will affect the relationship. Any time I start dating a guy, I feel that we have these invisible hurdles to cross before I can even think of a relationship with him. First, I have to find a way to tell him I had cancer. Then — if he's still around — I tell him I'm infertile. When I do, my whole body tenses up, bracing for the reaction. A lot of times that's the last I'll see of the guy. But usually before he splits, he will make a big point of wanting to be friends.

The way I look at it, I'll be very lucky if I ever find someone who will care for me enough to make it over those hurdles. I've reached the point where I'm okay with these issues, but a lot of people aren't. Most of the guys my age don't know what to say or how to act. I'm hoping all that will change once I get to graduate school, where people are older and hopefully more accepting.

In the meantime I've tried to take the negative things, refocus them, and then approach them as challenges. I'll tell myself, It's okay, Linda. So you can't have kids; it's not the end of the world. I mean, there are alternatives, like surrogacy or adoption. Just knowing that there are options helps me deal with it.

CANCER TREATMENT AND FEMALE INFERTILITY

Dramatic strides in the treatment of Hodgkin's disease mean that the vast majority of young people who are diagnosed with this type of cancer are living rather than dying. But for patients like Linda, the cure exacts the steep price of infertility.

In many ways, a woman's reproductive life is much more complex than that of her male counterpart. A man's testicles act very much like a twenty-four-hour semen factory, constantly producing new shipments of sperm. A woman, however, is born with a large but finite number of eggs (ova) in her ovaries, and that supply is slowly depleted throughout her reproductive life. Also, a woman's fertility is closely tied to her monthly menstrual cycle and the intricate hormonal commands that orchestrate it. Each month during ovulation, normally a single ovum is released from an ovary and begins its descent down the Fallopian tubes toward the uterus. It is during this journey that the egg is poised for a potential rendezvous with sperm — and possible fertilization.

It doesn't take much to disrupt the precise synchronization of a woman's reproductive cycle, and cancer treatment can deliver a powerful shock to the system. Chemotherapy will do this by interfering with a woman's hormone production, which

in turn interrupts the menstrual cycle, resulting in amenor-
rhea (suppressed menstrual period) or premature menopause.
Cyclophosphamide (Cytoxan), mechlorethamine (Mustar-
gen), chlorambucil (Leukeran), bulsulfan (Myleran), and vinblastine (Velban) are several chemo drugs known to interfere
with ovarian function and menstruation. In most cases this
side effect reverses itself once treatment is complete. Whether
these drugs cause permanent infertility or not usually depends
on the dose involved and the length of therapy. The more
aggressive and long-term chemotherapy is (as in Linda's case),
the more likely a woman is to experience fertility problems.

Age also plays a part in whether a woman's reproductive
system will bounce back from treatment. For example, younger women (aged twenty-five and under) who undergo chemotherapy treatment involving the drug Cytoxan will, in most
cases, eventually experience a return of their normal menstrual cycle, whereas women who are in their thirties and
early forties have a much greater chance of early menopause
and permanent sterility.

Dr. Phillip DiSaia is professor of obstetrics and gynecology
at the University of California–Irvine, where he holds the
Dorothy Marsh Chair in Reproductive Biology. A noted ex-
pert in the field of infertility, Dr. DiSaia explains why age plays
such an integral part in chemotherapy's effect on a woman's
ovaries.

If a woman is in her mid to late thirties, chemotherapy can in some
cases accelerate the depletion of whatever eggs she has left in her
reproductive life. But if treatment is lengthy or very intensive, it's
going to destroy all the remaining eggs. Keeping this in mind, an
oncologist will try to tailor his treatment plans accordingly and,
whenever possible, take appropriate preventative measures.

Dr. DiSaia adds that radiotherapy can also damage a woman's
reproductive capacity, although the extent of that risk de-

pends on the total dose and location of radiation as well as the age of the patient. For instance, radiation to a woman's pelvic area may interfere with her ability to have children if her treatment results in either ovarian failure or scarring of the vagina, uterus, or Fallopian tubes. Women who are at greatest risk for permanent infertility are those who receive full radiation to the pelvic area together with chemotherapy.

Oncologists are now developing innovative approaches to protect a patient's ovaries prior to treatment. A recent trend includes using briefer regimens of adjuvant chemotherapy. Experimental studies also suggest that for some patients the ovaries can be protected during chemotherapy by administering medication that temporarily halts ovulation. On another front, in a method similar to sperm banking, a technique known as ova retrieval allows women to freeze and store their eggs before they begin treatment. The frozen eggs can then be fertilized at a later date and implanted in the woman's uterus. Fertility may also be spared by using a technique known as ovarian transposition, which allows doctors to block or relocate a woman's ovaries surgically prior to radiation therapy. According to Dr. DiSaia:

By this method, the surgeon physically moves the ovaries, complete with their blood supply, outside of the area that is going to be irradiated. For example, with Hodgkin's patients, we will usually relocate a woman's ovaries by tacking them to the back of her uterus. This doesn't prevent the ovaries from functioning properly, it simply shields them from exposure. When radiation treatment is complete, the ovaries are then returned to their normal position. But the use of this procedure really depends on the type of cancer we are treating and where the radiation needs to be delivered.

In short, oncologists are taking steps to protect against the potential loss of a woman's childbearing ability, although options are limited by the type of cancer and how aggressively it needs to be treated. If you are faced with treatment that may affect your fertility, talk to your medical team and express whatever concerns you have. Find out what treatment options are open to you and what, if anything, your doctors can do to diminish damage to your reproductive system.

TESTING FOR INFERTILITY

Many women assume that since cancer treatment has interrupted their periods, they must be infertile. The fact that you aren't menstruating, however, doesn't mean you can't get pregnant. (And, needless to say, a woman undergoing cancer treatment should not try to become pregnant during or immediately after treatment.) If your period was interrupted by the effects of treatment, your doctor probably won't be able to tell you when or if it will return. However, there are several tests you can take to find out your fertility status. These tests include

- *Estradiol level test.* Estradiol is the most important of the estrogen hormones (female sex hormones) and can be used to measure the level of estrogen in your body. If treatment has resulted in total ovarian failure, estrogen will not be present in the bloodstream.
- *Serum FSH or LH test.* This test provides a more accurate indicator of ovarian dysfunction by measuring the amount of FSH (follicle stimulating hormone) and LH (luteinizing hormone) in the bloodstream. If these hormone levels are elevated, it can be a sign that both hormones are trying — albeit unsuccessfully — to stimulate ovulation.
- *Ovarian biopsy.* As a last resort, a doctor can perform this procedure to determine if you have any viable eggs left in your ovaries. The biopsy is performed surgically using a laparascope to remove a tiny sample from the outer layer of

an ovary. By studying this sample, your doctor can determine whether or not cancer treatment has actually destroyed all the eggs, resulting in complete ovarian failure. The procedure is painless and can be performed on an outpatient basis.

It is important to remember that for many women infertility is a temporary problem, even though it may take years to reverse itself. Unfortunately, doctors have no way of knowing who will experience a reversal; for some, it just never happens. However, these tests may clue you in on what's happening — or not happening — with your reproductive system.

Options for the Infertile Survivor

Should preliminary tests reveal that you are either infertile or subfertile or that treatment-related problems have made it impossible for you to carry a baby to term, don't give up hope. Astonishing advances in medical technology are enabling many more infertile people to have a biological child through such assisted reproductive techniques as *in vitro* fertilization and embryo transfer. But as sophisticated as these procedures are, they don't work for everyone. For some survivors, these options will prove to be undesirable, inappropriate, or unsuccessful, in which case they may consider adoption.

Should you opt to try for a biological child of your own, however, be sure to consult your gynecologist to help you decide which, if any, of the following assisted reproductive techniques might work for you.

ARTIFICIAL INSEMINATION BY HUSBAND (AIH)

Men who have either banked their sperm prior to treatment or who are experiencing subfertility as a result of their treatment can benefit from this procedure. With AIH, a man's sperm sample is deposited inside the woman's uterus at a time when she is known to be ovulating. Before performing this procedure, the doctor may medically process or "wash" the sperm sample to achieve better sperm concentration.

ARTIFICIAL INSEMINATION BY DONOR (AID)

In instances where the man is infertile and has no usable sperm sample, his mate may wish to undergo artificial insemination using sperm from an anonymous donor. The decision to use this method of conception is a highly personal one since the resulting embryo will not be biologically related to the father.

Since the outbreak of acquired immune deficiency syndrome (AIDS), infertile couples have voiced concern over the safety of donated sperm. You should know that sperm banks take stringent precautions to screen donor sperm for both genetic and sexually transmitted diseases. The American Fertility Society now recommends close monitoring and repeated testing of donor sperm for AIDS antibodies.

IN VITRO FERTILIZATION (IVF)

In vitro ("test-tube") fertilization no longer inhabits the brave new world of reproductive medicine; it is now, in fact, standard medical practice. In this procedure, eggs are removed from a woman's ovaries and mixed with a male's sperm sample in a laboratory dish. (In the early days of IVF, doctors used test tubes; hence the term *test-tube babies*.) If fertilization occurs, the resulting pre-embryo is placed back in the woman's uterus.

In theory IVF is easy, but in reality this form of treatment does not have a high success rate and requires a great deal of patience and commitment as well as a considerable financial commitment by the couple. Subfertile men may benefit from

IVF since with this method fewer sperm are needed to fertilize the egg. Even under auspicious laboratory conditions, however, fertilization will not occur if the sperm are abnormal or defective. Also, the woman's uterus must be functioning normally for the fertilized egg to implant successfully. Women who have experienced complete ovarian failure may choose to try IVF using donor eggs.

GAMETE INTRA-FALLOPIAN TRANSFER (GIFT) AND ZYGOTE INTRA-FALLOPIAN TRANSFER (ZIFT)

Both GIFT and ZIFT are variations of the IVF procedure. With GIFT, several ripened eggs are harvested from the woman's ovaries, quickly mixed with sperm in a catheter, and then immediately transferred back into the woman's Fallopian tube. If fertilization occurs, the rapidly dividing pre-embryo will then travel down the Fallopian tube to the uterus, where it may attach to the uterine lining. Because fertilization takes place within the woman's Fallopian tubes, the GIFT procedure can be said to come closest to duplicating natural conception.

In yet another variation known as zygote intra-Fallopian transfer, egg and sperm are first allowed to complete fertilization in a lab dish, and then the resulting pre-embryo is placed back into the woman's Fallopian tube. Candidates for either GIFT or ZIFT include men with low sperm counts and infertile women who choose to use donor eggs. Women who have blocked Fallopian tubes or damaged uteruses would not benefit from either of these procedures.

EMBRYO TRANSFER (DONOR EGGS)

What happens when cancer treatment causes a woman's ovaries to permanently shut down so that egg production and ovulation have ceased? Women who have been thrust by treatment into premature menopause have the option of using eggs donated by a close friend or relative. The donated egg is mixed with the sperm of the infertile woman's husband or mate and then transferred to her uterus or Fallopian tubes. Before the transfer is made, doctors use hormone therapy to "prime" the woman's uterus so that it will be receptive to the transplanted pre-embryo.

A major drawback to this method is the availability of donor eggs. Not every infertile woman has a relative or friend who is willing to donate eggs. The issue then becomes whether or not to use eggs from an anonymous donor. Donor eggs are available, but they are in limited supply.

SURROGACY

Hysterectomies and other forms of radical surgery to a woman's reproductive system almost always guarantee sterility. Women who have had hysterectomies can nevertheless still fulfill their hope of a biological child by "borrowing" the uterus of a close friend or relative. Two types of surrogacy exist. The first involves removing eggs from the sterile woman, provided of course that her ovaries are intact and producing healthy eggs. Her eggs are fertilized with her husband's sperm and the resulting pre-embryo is then transferred to the surrogate mother's uterus. If the procedure is successful, the surrogate will carry the infertile couple's baby to term.

In another form of surrogacy, the surrogate's own eggs are artificially inseminated with the sperm of the husband or mate of the infertile woman. The surrogate then surrenders the baby to the infertile couple at birth.

Surrogacy is an extraordinarily complex and controversial topic, and events such as the highly publicized case of Baby M have raised a storm of legal and ethical questions regarding its practice. Survivors considering this option should be fully aware of the potential legal and emotional ramifications.

Will you find success using one of these methods? That depends on a variety of factors, including your age and overall health, the cause of your infertility, and the quality of the sperm sample and its ability to fertilize an egg. Should you decide to use a procedure that includes the biological participation of someone other than you and your mate (as with surrogacy, procedures using donor eggs, or AID), be sure to first consult a lawyer or social worker who is knowledgeable about the legal issues involved. You and your partner also need to weigh the emotional issues attached to these methods and discuss how your feelings will affect your relationship now and in the future.

Also, you should understand that these techniques are expensive, time-consuming, and emotionally exhausting. On top of that, virtually all of them have a low success rate. If you plan to go ahead with infertility treatment, bear in mind that these procedures offer hope to some, not guarantees for all.

The Challenge of Adoption

What happens when these assisted reproductive technologies fail, when all hope of having a biological child disappears? The most difficult time for infertile couples comes when they must face the hard, cold medical facts of infertility and acknowledge that their dream of having a child must now be reconciled with reality. The infertile couple need to reshape their expectations around a different notion of parenthood, one that may include thoughts of adoption.

It is not easy to face up to the idea of adoption. Before you can even think of moving on to this "second choice," you'll need to come to terms with your loss of fertility and resolve the emotions that loss has engendered. It also means sorting out how you really feel about adoption.

For many infertile couples, adoption means fully acknowledging the idea that the infant they bring home will not be genetically related to either partner. It also means accepting the possibility that even this alternative to parenting may ultimately elude them. But for those who do succeed in adopting, the joy of finally having a child to call their own can be overwhelming, and the rewards endless.

For survivors of cancer, however, the issue of adoption is a lot more prickly. Because of their medical history, recovered patients run a higher than average risk of being rejected by traditional adoption agencies. That risk, together with the long and emotionally taxing trip through the adoption maze, is enough to discourage even the most sanguine survivor from even thinking about adoption. One Cancervive member underscored this point when she said:

For me, dealing with the fear of rejection and the sense of isolation it brings is one of the challenges of being a survivor. When I realize the risks I'd be taking by going through the adoption process, I'd just as soon not stick my neck out. It's much easier not having to deal with yet another round of rejection.

Michael Hubner of Boston's Beth Israel Hospital comments on the hesitation infertile survivors feel when their thoughts turn to adoption:

For those who have already experienced cancer treatment and infertility, leaving themselves open to that kind of emotional loss all over again is even more devastating than it would be for the normal infertile person. You desperately want the chance to adopt a child, and yet you also want to spare yourself any further loss or injury to self-esteem. It is these two conflicting desires that can paralyze a survivor's attempt at adoption.

The process of adopting through traditional agencies can be fraught with frustration. As an alternative, many survivors turn to private adoption, in which the couple deal directly with the birth mother or through an intermediary such as a lawyer or doctor. But survivors and social workers have informed me that, in some ways, private adoption comes with its own set of pitfalls. For instance, private adoption tends to cost much more than traditional adoptions. Then again, like other infertile people, survivors run the risk of having the birth mother renege on her promise to surrender the baby.

Of course, not every survivor who chooses adoption faces certain rejection. The criteria adoption agencies use to screen applicants vary widely from state to state, although the basic requirements are fairly standard. For example, adoption agencies consider only couples who are in "stable relationships," that is, those who have been married for several years and who have what the agency regards as sound financial and social backgrounds. Most traditional agencies will not even consider divorced or single persons. Your date of birth also comes into play; agencies generally regard age forty as the cut-off point for eligibility.

But for survivors, the real stumbling block to adoption lies in the medical history requirement. Many have found that the adoption process comes to a screeching halt once the word *cancer* is mentioned. Even long-term survivors say that they have a hard time convincing either the agency or the birth mother that they are indeed disease-free, even though their physicians have confirmed it in writing.

"Certain agencies are going to systematically reject an application based on a cancer history," says Eli Lefferman. "I think it's wrong, but that's what they do." Dr. Lefferman is director of community services at Vista Del Mar Child and Family Services in Los Angeles, a multiservice family agency on the cutting edge of adoption-related issues. He stresses that it is the agency's responsibility to make sure that the birth mother is fully informed about the health status of each of the applicants. He emphasizes, however, that it is the birth mother who ultimately makes the final decision regarding to whom she relinquishes her baby.

Where does that leave you? Isn't it likely that the stigma still associated with cancer will demolish your chances? Dr. Lefferman responds:

Sometimes that happens. That is one of the reasons why it is so essential for you, as an applicant with a cancer history, to get a letter from your doctor describing the state of your health and your long-term prognosis. But it is equally important for you and your spouse to meet with the birth mother as soon as possible and try to connect with her on a personal level. It's probably not a good idea to tell her about your cancer history during that first meeting. Let her get to know you first. Then perhaps by the second or third meeting, you can bring it up so the three of you can discuss it.

Survivors of cancer, or for that matter any life-threatening disease, shouldn't feel shut out of the adoption process. I wouldn't say you have just as much chance as everyone else, but that doesn't mean you have absolutely no chance, either. I know of several survivors who have successfully adopted. In most instances, it happens because the birth mother connected to the couple's medical problem. Perhaps the birth mother has a friend or relative who has survived cancer, and so she is familiar with the issues involved. Or perhaps she realized that, because of their life-threatening experience, the adoptive parents now have a heightened appreciation of life. And that may be precisely the kind of people she is looking for to raise her child.

According to Dr. Lefferman, the most important signal a survivor can send to an adoption agency or birth mother is one of hope and confidence. But if unresolved emotions are still churning inside you, they may undermine your confidence and affect how you present yourself. This is why it's so important to come to terms with your infertility (and, if you

haven't already, your cancer experience) before you even begin to think about adoption.

   Ellen Glazer is a licensed clinical social worker in private
practice in Boston. She is the author of *The Long-Awaited Stork:
A Guide Book for Parents After Infertility* (Lexington Books, 1990)
and co-author of *Without Child: Experiencing and Resolving
Infertility* (Lexington Books, 1988). In addition, Glazer also
serves as a member of the board of Resolve, a national infertility support group. She offers cancer survivors this advice
on adoption:

- *Minimize your vulnerability.* Adoption agencies will ask for a
  letter from your physician regarding your condition. If you
  know that it is too soon for your doctor to be able to write a
  thoroughly optimistic letter, perhaps you are better off waiting. This may be difficult, especially if you and your partner
  are getting older or have been waiting for a long time to become parents.
- *Remember that for you, approval for adoption is an important confirmation that others believe in your health and in your future.* Try
  to keep this issue in mind. It will help you understand why
  you find the adoption process especially stressful — and
  why you feel like so much is riding on it.
- *Come to terms with the honesty issue.* Some adoptive parents and
  some agencies insist that honesty is always the best policy
  when it comes to adoption. However, I am aware of instances in which couples chose not to disclose their cancer
  history and have successfully adopted. Try to determine
  what is in the best interest of the child and act on it.
- *Choose a low-risk adoption.* Given all that you have been
  through, try to select an adoption that involves a minimum
  of risk. Avoid adoptions that may fall through (such as open
  adoptions), babies that might be seriously ill, and any legally
  risky situations. Such precautions may require more time or

money on your part. But in the long run this will be less painful than putting yourself in situations in which you may face further loss.

• *Distinguish minimal risk from expediency.* Remember that adoption is a lifetime commitment to a complete stranger. It would be a big mistake to undertake a particular type of adoption because it appears less complicated. Couples should be especially cautious about adopting an older or hard-to-adopt child. It is easy to develop "rescue fantasies" when you are thinking about adoption, but it is very hard to live with a child who has gone through difficult times. Don't talk yourself into this kind of adoption because you think it will be easy; it won't.

• *Recognize the difference between adoption and biological reproduction.* Finally, it is important for all adopting parents, and especially those who have survived cancer, to fully acknowledge the fact that adoptive parenting is different from biological parenting. Although there are many aspects of parenting that have nothing to do with birth or adoption, it does feel different to parent a child who was not born to you. In order to successfully adopt and delight in your new child, you must have mourned the lost potential for your own biological offspring. After your struggle with cancer, this loss is, indeed, a double blow.

ALTERNATIVES TO ADOPTION

For survivors who don't qualify for adoption, surrogacy (for females) and donor insemination (for males) are the remaining options to parenthood. As controversial as these alternatives are, infertile survivors often find them less ambiguous and uncertain than adoption. They are no less emotionally complicated, however. You and your mate need to ask yourselves what it will mean to raise a child who will be biologically related to only one of you. And can you accept having a child through a procedure that is not yet considered socially secure? Before you decide to pursue these parenting alternatives, be sure to examine all the ethical, emotional, and legal issues involved.

Then again, not every infertile person is eager to become a parent. Some survivors elect to remain childless. For these people, life without children makes perfect sense; it fits their lifestyle and plans for the future. Contrary to what society tells us, children aren't necessarily a requisite for happiness and self-fulfillment. It all depends on your outlook. When feminist Gloria Steinem, herself a survivor of breast cancer, was asked why she decided not to have children, she replied, "I had a choice: I either gave birth to someone else, or I gave birth to myself."

The Emotions of Infertility

How will you react when tests reveal that your infertility is untreatable? You've tried everything medical science has to offer, with no success. The results are back, the prognosis is in.

You are permanently sterile.

Even though you may have suspected it, your doctor's words still come as a terrible shock, a palpable blow. Once you've absorbed this information, you may find initial feelings of shock melting into denial or anger. You know the reaction. You'll hear yourself saying, "This isn't happening to me! I *can't* be sterile!" For some people, this news is just too painful, too threatening to their self-esteem and security. So they protect themselves by rejecting it, or by pretending that their infertility is only a temporary problem. For most people, denial serves as the first line of defense against a crisis, and the crisis of infertility is handled no differently. Survivors who were never told their treatment might lead to sterility frequently have the most trouble accepting the news; their first reaction of shock and surprise is mixed with a deep sense of distrust and betrayal.

According to Christine Perkins, Cancervive's director of social services, denial plays an important part in allowing the mind to adjust slowly to the news of infertility.

Like a psychic Band-Aid, denial can protect you during the time you are most vulnerable. But sooner or later you'll need to get past denial so that you can heal completely. That can only take place once you've allowed yourself to work through all the other emotions involved in the grieving process, emotions that your denial may be suppressing.

Grieving will give you the opportunity to rework your self-image so that your sexuality and self-esteem are no longer so dependent on whether or not you can have children. You will discover that regardless of your infertility, you can be comfortable with who you are and content with what you have to offer the world.

But many survivors become stuck in the denial stage, unwilling or unable to relinquish their dream of having children. They choose to continue harboring the hope that somehow they will be different, that one day soon they will confound the odds, surprise the doctors, and succeed in having a baby. But as years go by and the reality of infertility sinks in, their denial may suddenly and unexpectedly give way to anger and resentment.

If that happens to you, don't be alarmed. Again, this is a normal response to the loss you feel. Says Perkins, "Anger is an important part of the grieving process; it compels you to react to what you perceive to be the injustice of your infertility."

Like Kevin and Linda, you may find yourself projecting

your anger onto those you believe to be most responsible: your parents, the oncologist, God, yourself. You may also find that getting beyond the blame and resentment isn't easy. Michael Hubner says that the anger survivors feel is much more complicated than the anger felt by other infertile people:

It's a strange sort of blunted anger, because you're angry at the people who made the decision to save your life. It's not a clear-cut emotion, and certainly not easy to resolve. As a result, you may feel guilty over the way you are feeling. Also, society keeps telling you that you should be grateful to be alive. But that's not always possible, because you have experienced great loss, and it undermines any feeling you have of gratitude.

In addition, your anger may be a reaction to the loss of control that both cancer and infertility represent. As a survivor, you already live with a heightened sense of vulnerability, an unsettling realization that your body, once so self-sufficient and reliable, doesn't always work the way it should. Adds Hubner:

You want children, but your body won't cooperate. You long to live to a ripe old age, yet cancer seems to shadow you, forever threatening your chances. Life is unpredictable, full of disappointment and unanticipated loss. Cancer tells you that and infertility confirms it. But it's certainly not impossible to transcend those challenges and find meaning, fulfillment, and happiness in life.

Still, survivors point out that infertility, like cancer, sets them apart; they often feel alienated from their peers, even from other infertile people. Like Linda, many single survivors who are infertile worry about dating and establishing close relationships. They see themselves as biological failures, outcasts from the gene pool, and therefore undesirable to the opposite sex. To minimize the risk of rejection, they may choose instead to date only other infertile people. But that doesn't always work either. One reason is that infertile people who are not survivors often have more reproductive options open to them. Then again, many of them can't understand the profound sense of isolation that the double blow of cancer and infertility represents to survivors.

In fact, some survivors become so sensitized to the issue of infertility that they go out of their way to avoid people and social events that may remind them of it. Linda says that for several years she had trouble socializing with girlfriends who were either pregnant or new mothers.

I remember going to my best friend's shower two years after I'd learned about my infertility. I thought I could handle it, that I was beyond all the heavy emotions. But I felt so envious and angry at the shower that I left early and cried all the way home. Since then I've stayed away from baby showers and birthdays. I used to think that in time it would get easier for me to accept my infertility, but there seems to be a part of me that still hasn't come to terms with it. Baby showers and birth announcements are supposed to be joyful occasions, but for me they are just another painful reminder.

Like Linda, you may have trouble fully accepting your infertility, and as a consequence it could be affecting other parts of your life. Failure or inability to grieve over infertility can stem from a variety of reasons. A sense of guilt — over the anger you are feeling, or because you think infertility is somehow your fault — could be blocking the grieving process. You may feel that grieving over infertility isn't quite legitimate or socially acceptable. Perhaps you don't perceive your loss as real. After all, you might think, no one actually died. That's true; there are no funerals, no tombstones for the unconceived. The loss you feel is less tangible than the death of a loved one, but in its own way it's just as profound. Infertility marks the passing of a dream. It represents the very real loss of genetic continuity made possible by biological children. That, notes Hubner, is the tragic irony, the terrible paradox, at the heart of treatment-induced infertility. And it is perhaps the most difficult aspect to accept:

As human beings, we are forever looking for ways of becoming immortal, of extending ourselves either biologically or metaphorically into the future, so that we can leave something of ourselves behind. In this way, children become our images of immortality; they represent life replenished. But while cancer treatment may extend your life, it is at the cost of having future children.

The emotions of infertility are very personal and complex as well as puzzling and painful. You may not be able to resolve your grief alone — and you shouldn't feel that you have to. Infertility is a life crisis shared by millions of people, some of them survivors. Because of the nature of cancer treatment, the National Cancer Institute estimates that infertility is 15 percent more common among survivors than among other adults. In short, you are not alone.

But you may be uncertain of how to reach out for help. One important source of emotional support is Resolve, the national nonprofit organization for infertile people. This Boston-based organization has been offering infertility counseling, referrals, and support to members since 1973. With the help and support of groups like Resolve and the healing powers of time, faith, and optimism, many infertile people have learned how to accept and integrate infertility into their lives. Call your local chapter of Resolve for information about group meetings or to learn about other Resolve members in your area who are also cancer survivors. Resolve is located at 5 Water Street, Arlington, Mass. 02174 (tel. 800-662-1016).

Remember that when all is said and done, infertility doesn't change who you are. You still have the capacity to love, to create, to appreciate life and leave your mark on the world. It took me many years, as well as counseling and the support of my husband, before I could fully accept my own infertility.

Learn to let go of your loss and find ways to feel good about yourself. It may help if you can come to view your infertility in a positive light. Cancer treatment may have taken away your ability to have children, but it has given you the gift of life. It's a bittersweet victory, but a victory nonetheless.

Paving the Way

In many ways, today's recovered cancer patients are much more than just survivors. Rather, they are like trailblazers, clearing a wilderness of survivorship issues, paving a path for others to follow. They are doing this by speaking up about such long-term effects issues as treatment-caused infertility and expressing how these issues affect the quality of survival. They are clearing the way for future patients by drawing attention to patients' rights and by demanding more informed consent. Doctors are in turn responding by providing additional information, seeking less toxic therapies, and doing what they can to minimize reproductive damage. But, as Michael Hubner notes, much more needs to be done:

Even though cancer survival rates have improved, there is still no vocal constituency of survivors who are speaking up and telling the medical community, "Look at us. We are surviving five, ten — even thirty years or more after diagnosis. And infertility is one of the many issues we are still struggling with." Survivors need to organize just like any other advocacy group and demand change. They have to focus attention on the issue of infertility and continue raising the consciousness of health care providers by asking "Why wasn't I told?" and "Why aren't there any real alternatives?"

That message came across loud and clear when, at a recent Cancervive meeting, a member noted, "When you think about it, we're all part of a transitional generation. Twenty-five years ago, none of us would have been lucky enough to be sitting around talking about infertility."

Linda was at that meeting. She replied by saying, "But you know what? In ten years, there will be another group of people sitting here who will have survived cancer with their fertility intact. And it will be because of people like us."

10

Cancervive

THIS BOOK began with a journey. It is only fitting that it should end with a look at where that journey has led, and the discoveries I made along the way.

Since our initial support group meeting in 1985, my co-founder Lisa and I realized how much the burgeoning survivor population needed an organization like Cancervive. It filled a void in cancer care previously overlooked by the medical community.

The challenge both exhilarated and intimidated us. But propelled by our emotional commitment, we plunged headlong into fulfilling our dream without really knowing how to make it a working reality. After all, how did one go about setting up a nonprofit organization? What kind of programs should we offer? How would we raise the funds to support our activities?

"We just *do* it," said Lisa matter-of-factly when I called her in San Francisco to report the success of the first few meetings. "We'll do what we can and we'll ask for help when we need it. And I promise, as soon as I can escape from this hospital, I'll be there to give you a hand."

Lisa's enthusiasm and desire to help belied her physical condition; the long-term complications of treatment were continuing to take their toll on her. The hospital was now her primary place of residence as she underwent innumerable medical procedures. Her input and participation in Cancervive became limited to talks on the phone from her hospital bed.

Lisa's plight spurred me on. Five hundred miles south in Los Angeles, I began putting together Cancervive's board of directors and organizing more support group meetings. With the financial and emotional support of my parents, I quit my job and dedicated myself full-time to our fledgling organization. I set up a makeshift office in my apartment and was on the phone every day talking to media people, hospital administrators, and oncology social workers.

Fund-raising was of course a constant concern, and Lisa and I plotted ways of ferreting out financial support. Help would often appear unsolicited. An acquaintance offered to provide us with her services as a public relations consultant. A local firm donated a personal computer. A typesetting shop owned by a cancer survivor offered to prepare our newsletter free of charge. Little miracles like this assured me that Cancervive was going to make it.

With the help of two social workers, I set down the organization's basic philosophy. We decided that a person must be disease-free and off treatment at least six months before joining a Cancervive support group. Initially, many people questioned my insistence on this point. They asked, Isn't anyone with a cancer diagnosis essentially a survivor? I didn't think so. In my view, the cancer patient and the survivor are at two distinctly different developmental stages. I knew this from my own experience, and the many health professionals I spoke to concurred with my view. As a survivor, my needs and concerns were centered around the challenges of life *after* cancer — issues related to the disease but as distinct from the patient stage as spring from winter.

I also wanted Cancervive to serve as a sort of lightship to guide recovered patients once they had navigated their way through treatment and were headed back into the mainstream. I remember taking a call from a woman who had recently been diagnosed with leukemia. She was interested in attending one of our support groups. I explained to her the criterion for joining Cancervive and then gave her a number of referrals to patient-oriented support groups. I hung up the phone feeling vaguely depressed, as if I'd somehow let her down. Two days later I received a large donation in the mail. To my surprise, it was from the woman with leukemia. Along with the check, she included a note: "This is to assure that Cancervive will be there for me once I become a survivor."

Within a few months, my two telephone lines were swamped with calls from people wanting to know more about the organization. As word spread, our support groups multiplied. By 1986 I'd hired a social worker to head a second chapter of Cancervive in the nearby San Fernando Valley. The feedback from those who attended our meetings was phenomenal.

"It helps so much to hash out my problems with people who can identify with them," said one woman. Another person observed, "At other cancer support groups, I always felt that, as a survivor, I was supposed to serve as the 'example' to group members who were still fighting the disease. At Cancervive I don't have to worry about putting on a front." Someone else said simply, "I'm so relieved to know I'm not alone."

Lisa was delighted to hear about the groundswell of support Cancervive was receiving. "We've finally found our oasis in the desert!" she cheered. Our dream was now a tangible reality.

To my surprise, Cancervive was having a powerful effect on me as well. I had been so busy with the nuts and bolts of running a nonprofit organization that I was slow to realize how my involvement in it was changing my life. I felt as if I'd finally reached a point where I could be who I really was and share my experience in a positive way with other people.

Of course, that kind of self-acceptance didn't arrive overnight. Instead it was a gradual, evolutionary process. One particular incident sticks in my mind as the turning point. I was on a flight returning from Washington, D.C., where I had attended a conference on issues facing survivors. The flight was crowded, and I was exhausted. To make matters worse, my right leg was swollen and sore. I couldn't have been doing a very good job of hiding my discomfort because the man sitting next to me turned and asked if something was wrong. My first impulse was to discount my leg and pretend that I was fine. But something made me stop and think, Why should I lie? What do I have to hide? Instead, I told him that cancer treatment for my leg many years ago had resulted in a chronic swelling problem.

"You mean you have lymphedema?" he asked. "Wouldn't it help if you elevated it? Here, use my knee to prop up your leg."

I was pleasantly surprised by his openness and concern, and with a grateful smile took him up on the offer. As it turned out, he was married to a woman who also had lymphedema. He explained that his wife's condition was the result of a radical mastectomy. We talked about cancer, my organization, and the issues of survivorship all the way to Los Angeles. On that flight I made up my mind to "come clean" with my cancer history. I no longer felt the need to lie to strangers or cloak my disabled leg in alibis.

The layers of protection I'd used all those years to insulate myself began to fall away, and in the process my personal life grew more fulfilling. Best of all was my deepening relationship with Steve Nessim, a good friend I'd known since high school. Steve had always been there in my own backyard, so to speak, but I'd never really noticed him before. He believed in what I wanted to achieve with Cancervive and was my most ardent supporter. In fact, Steve was Cancervive's first contributor, presenting me with a check for $1,018. The extra eighteen dollars, he explained, was symbolic. The number stands for *chai* — Hebrew for "life."

Steve feels that our marriage in 1986 was largely made possible by Cancervive. He knew that until I'd resolved my deep feelings of anger and frustration we wouldn't work as a couple.

He was right. I know now that survivors need to make peace with what has happened to them. Until we learn to make the experience a positive and constructive force in our lives, our relationships will always be loaded down by the emotional baggage left over from cancer. That's certainly how it was for me.

One of my favorite poems, "Don't Ask," by the Chilean poet Pablo Neruda, refers to a person who is forever lugging around a sack of stones. Each of us, in our own way, carries around a cache of stones. You either learn to be comfortable carrying around those stones, or you find a way to lay them aside. Survivors need a place to unburden themselves of fear, anger, and sadness. That, quite simply, is the reason for Cancervive.

In my view, that's also the significance of all support groups. They give us a sense of security, a safe haven, a collective atmosphere of caring and support. Shared experience is the glue that forms an instant bond between members — a sort of camaraderie of the campfire. In that sense, a support group can provide the kind of psychological salve that promotes healing. It is also an effective antidote to the isolation, the sense of aloneness, that is so much a part of cancer's terrain.

At a recent support meeting, I asked several Cancervive members to discuss what they had gained from belonging to the group.

JEREMY: Cancervive is different from any other support group I've attended. Other groups included people who were still in treatment. They were in the middle of that intense, fight-for-your-life stage. How could I talk about my problems as a survivor when in comparison my worries seemed so insignificant? But here I feel like I can be open about what's really bothering me.

NORA: As a survivor, I now find I have the emotional distance to make sense of what happened to me as a patient. Talking to other survivors helps me put it in perspective and distill from it all kinds of insights. It becomes a process of healing.

JESSE: I appreciate that Cancervive support groups don't meet in a hospital setting. My group meets in a hotel conference room, and for me, it's much more relaxing that way. There's something about meeting in a hospital that puts me in a "patient" state of mind, and I don't see myself in that role anymore. As it is, it's depressing enough having to go back to the hospital for checkups.

LENA: My marriage broke up several months after my treatment for melanoma. When I first came to the group I wasn't sure I would ever make sense of what had happened. To my surprise, I found myself crying in front of total strangers. They knew the kind of confusion and pain I was feeling in a way none of my friends could. This group has been my emotional anchor.

CLAUDIA: Even though I have a very loving and supportive family, they can't really understand what I've gone through — and that's a lonely feeling. I imagine it's the way combat veterans feel when they come home from war, or survivors of airplane crashes. The experience has made you part of a special group — those who have "been there." You come away from it with a different view of life.

ANITA: People always think that once treatment ends, a cancer patient's life magically falls back into place. But I think that's the rare exception. In many ways, being a survivor is much harder than being a patient. That's when the isolation sets in, and the fear of recurrence. A survivor support group is really a first-line defense against that.

PAUL (*to Anita*): I know what you mean. But it wasn't easy for me to understand at first. It took me a while to accept that I might feel better talking about cancer. For me, it was the whole macho thing — grin and bear it. During my recovery, my family didn't want to hear about cancer anymore. And they certainly didn't want me talking about what might happen if I got a recurrence. I took their cue and started denying a lot of what I was really feeling. But fear of recurrence has been the big hurdle for me, and that was tough facing by myself. When it started getting the better of me, I decided I needed to do something. The first few support group meetings I went to I didn't say a word. Now they practically have to tell me to shut up.

MELANIE: That's just it! In a support group you can let it all hang out, really be yourself — not someone you think others want you to be. It's a safe place to raise issues you can't verbalize anywhere else. For instance, no one wants to hear me talk about being infertile. But at Cancervive, I can really open up about a lot of stuff that's bothering me without someone judging me.

LINDA: One of the great things about a group like Cancervive is that I can learn from other people's coping techniques. After I found out that my chemo-related hearing problems would be permanent, I had all of this anger inside me. At a meeting, I heard Jeremy mention that when he gets upset he shuts himself in a room and screams it out. That kind of therapy had never occurred to me before. I decided to try it. I got in my car one night, drove out to a deserted spot, turned the radio up high, and started screaming my lungs out. I kept it up until I was completely exhausted. And you know what? It really helped. The only trouble is that whenever I do it, I have to keep an eye out for the cops. It's kind of embarrassing having to explain my "primal scream" therapy to them.

The reasons for joining a Cancervive support group are as diverse as the individuals who attend them. But two common bonds unite these people: a history of cancer and the desire to talk about it with other survivors. Talk may be cheap — but don't overlook its curative powers. There's something wonderfully reassuring about hearing how fellow survivors have handled the dark demons of fear and anger, guilt and depression. Peer-to-peer support may be good for your physical health as well. Researchers at Stanford University and the University of California–Berkeley have discovered that cancer patients who receive emotional and social support through group therapy tend to survive up to twice as long as patients who rely on medical treatment alone. Communication, it would seem, is not only therapeutic but life-giving as well.

At the heart of every survivor support group is a celebration of life, stripped of its materialistic trappings, pared down to an elegant understanding of what it means to be alive. A cancer diagnosis splashes you with a sort of ontological awareness, and survival hones that awareness into a steely-edged wisdom. People who have recovered from cancer savor life as only survivors can.

Of course, not everyone is comfortable being a "groupie" — and that's okay too. Some survivors have told me that they don't respond well to what they perceive as the "touchie-feelie" nature of support groups. Others say they have trouble coping with other people's problems; it compounds their own pain and suffering. Then again, some people just prefer to keep their emotions private. For these people there are always other options such as individual therapy, meditation, or prayer, to name just a few.

But if you haven't visited a support group, I suggest you give it a try. Survivors who appear to gain the most from group therapy are individuals who have decided to accept cancer as part of their identity and want to integrate the experience. In my years with Cancervive I've noticed that survivors often come to this decision at different times in their lives.

For instance, three years ago a young woman, a survivor of osteogenic sarcoma (bone cancer), came to her first Cancervive meeting. She said very little at the meeting, offering only that during her treatment doctors had performed a limb salvage procedure to save her leg. Afterward she approached me and inquired about my limp. As we walked out to our cars together I told her about my cancer treatment and how I had dealt with its repercussions. We parted ways, and she didn't come back. I concluded that Cancervive simply didn't offer the kind of help she was looking for. But several months ago, that same woman resurfaced and has been attending meetings on a regular basis ever since. She admitted that seeing me limp at that first meeting terrified her because doctors had told her that one day she might have trouble walking as a result of her treatment. Three years ago she hadn't been ready to accept that; now she was. I know that it wasn't easy for her to get to that point. A decade ago, I too began the same process of taking stock. And I learned that sometimes beginning the journey is as important as arriving at the destination.

As of this writing there are eight Cancervive chapters, seven in California and one in Texas, with others soon to be established around the country. Each chapter offers private and group counseling led by licensed clinical social workers and psychologists. In addition, Cancervive provides telephone counseling, a quarterly newsletter, and advocacy on behalf of survivor issues.

There are currently six million survivors of cancer in the United States. That's a lot of people — a potent constituency. Many of the important issues facing survivors — employment discrimination, insurance problems, biomedical issues related to cancer treatment — are slowly attracting national attention.

But more needs to be done. While the camaraderie of other survivors may be our greatest source of comfort and support, education and advocacy are our greatest weapons against fear and discrimination. We need to band together to make a difference.

Lisa and I started Cancervive with the hope that through our organization and others like it we could chip away at cancer's stubborn stigma and the barriers it creates. It is my desire that survivors will one day feel proud of having had cancer, and that others will come to regard it, in the words of Dr. Fitzhugh Mullan, as "a gritty badge of distinction." Lisa and I always felt that because of our cancer we had something special to offer the world — an alertness to life's nuances, a keener insight into others, a resiliency and strength that comes from having stared down death and faced up to the battle.

Lisa's own battle ended on August 14, 1988. During her final months in the hospital she did her best to convince me that her condition wasn't as serious as it seemed. I used to say she had nine lives, but this time I knew I was losing her. If nothing else, I wanted Cancervive to stand for Lisa's long, brave struggle. To me, her courage, determination, and vitality exemplified what it means to be a survivor.

I never got the chance to say goodbye to Lisa, but there isn't a day that goes by that I don't feel her presence. It's there at every support group meeting in the sharing and support, the empathy and the acceptance.

Surviving cancer is an experience wrought with pain, joy, anger, and optimism. It challenges our ability to endure. By sifting through our losses and gains, by accepting and letting go, we seek not just to endure but to thrive. And for survivors, that's the riskiest and noblest challenge of all.

BIBLIOGRAPHY

The American Cancer Society Cancer Book. Ed. Arthur I. Holleb, M.D. et al. New York: Doubleday, 1986.

American Cancer Society. *Cancer: Your Job, Insurance, and the Law.* Bull. no. 84-100M-4585-PS, 1984.

Andrieu, Jean Marie, M.D., and Maria Elena Ochoa-Molina. "Menstrual Cycle, Pregnancies and Offspring Before and After MOPP Therapy for Hodgkin's Disease." *Cancer* 52 (1983): 435–438.

Beisser, Arnold R., M.D. "Denial and Affirmation in Illness and Health." *American Journal of Psychiatry* 136 (August 1979): 1026–1030.

Beller, Sam E., with William Proctor. *The Great Insurance Secret.* New York: William Morrow, 1988.

Benjamin, Harold H. *From Victim to Victor.* Los Angeles: Tarcher, 1987.

Bentley, Judith. *The National Health Care Controversy.* New York: Franklin Watts, 1981.

Broyard, Anatole. "Doctor, Talk to Me." *New York Times Magazine,* August 26, 1990.

———. "Intoxicated by My Illness." *New York Times Magazine,* November 12, 1989.

Bruning, Nancy. *Coping with Chemotherapy.* New York: Doubleday, 1985.

Butler, Francelia. *Cancer Through the Ages.* Fairfax: Virginia Press, 1955.

Cassileth, Barrie R., Ph.D., et al. *The Cancer Patient.* Ed. Barrie R. Cassileth, Ph.D. Philadelphia: Lea & Febiger, 1979.

Chesler, Mark A., and Oscar A. Barbarin. *Childhood Cancer and the Family.* New York: Brunner/Mazel, 1987.

Christ, Grace A. "Social Consequences of the Cancer Experience." *American Journal of Pediatric Hematology/Oncology* 9 (1987): 84–88.

Clark, Matt, with Holly Morris et al. "Learning to Survive." *Newsweek*, April 8, 1985.

Cousins, Norman. *Anatomy of an Illness*. New York: Norton, 1979.

———. *Head First*. New York: Dutton, 1989.

Crothers, Helen. "Health Insurance: Problems and Solutions for People with Cancer Histories." American Cancer Society, *Proceedings of the Fifth National Conference on Human Values and Cancer*, San Francisco (1987): 100–109.

Dackman, Linda. *Up Front: Sex and the Post-Mastectomy Woman*. New York: Viking, 1990.

Davidson, Glen W. *Understanding Mourning: A Guide for Those Who Grieve*. Minneapolis: Augsburg, 1984.

Dietz, J. Herbert, Jr., M.D. *Rehabilitation Oncology*. New York: Wiley, 1981.

Dobkin, Patricia, and Gary R. Morrow, Ph.D. "Long-Term Side Effects in Patients Who Have Been Successfully Treated for Cancer." *Journal of Psychosocial Oncology* 3 (Winter 1985/86): 23–51.

Downie, Patricia A. *Cancer Rehabilitation*. London: Faber & Faber, 1976.

Dubquet, Virginia. "Overview of Reasonable Accommodation." *Access to Employment*, Winter 1984.

Feldman, Frances L. "Wellness and Work." In *Psychosocial Stress and Cancer*, ed. C. L. Cooper. New York: Wiley, 1984.

Fiore, Neil A. *The Road Back to Health*. New York: Bantam, 1984.

Fishman, Steve. "Cancer Comes Home." *New York Times Magazine*, June 11, 1989.

Gogan, Janis L., et al. "Pediatric Cancer Survival and Marriage: Issues Affecting Adult Adjustment." *American Journal of Orthopsychiatry* 49 (July 1979): 423–430.

Goldberg, Richard J., M.D., and Robert M. Tull, Ph.D. *The Psychosocial Dimensions of Cancer*. New York: Macmillan, 1983.

Goodman, Ellen. *Turning Points*. New York: Fawcett Columbine, 1979.

Graham, Jory. *In the Company of Others*. New York: Harcourt Brace Jovanovich, 1982.

Green, Daniel M., M.D. *Long-Term Complications of Therapy for Cancer in Childhood and Adolescence*. Baltimore: Johns Hopkins University Press, 1989.

Greenberg, Mimi, Ph.D. *Invisible Scars*. New York: Walker, 1988.

Hamilton, Joan O. C. "The Prognosis on Health Care: Critical — and Getting Worse." *Business Week*, January 9, 1989.

Hendin, Herbert, and Ann Pollinger Haas. *Wounds of War*. New York: Basic Books, 1984.

Hoffman, Barbara. "Cancer Survivors at Work: Job Problems and Illegal Discrimination." *Oncology Nursing Forum* 16 (January/February 1989): 39–43.

Holland, Jimmie C., Ph.D., and Julia H. Rowland, Ph.D., eds. *Handbook of Psychooncology*. New York: Oxford University Press, 1989.

Johnson, Judi L., R.N., Ph.D., and Linda Klein. *I Can Cope: Staying Healthy with Cancer*. Minneapolis: DCI Publishing, 1988.

Kalter, Suzy. *Looking Up*. New York: McGraw-Hill, 1987.

Kauffman, Danette G. *Surviving Cancer*. Washington, D.C.: Acropolis, 1987.

Kleinman, Arthur, M.D. *The Illness Narratives*. New York: Basic Books, 1988.

Koocher, Gerald P., Ph.D., and John E. O'Malley, M.D. *The Damocles Syndrome*. New York: McGraw-Hill, 1981.

Koocher, Gerald P., et al. "Psychological Adjustment Among Pediatric Cancer Survivors." *Journal of Child Psychology and Psychiatry* 21 (1980): 163–173.

Kopp, Sheldon. *Raise Your Right Hand Against Fear*. Minneapolis: CompCare, 1988.

Kübler-Ross, Elisabeth, M.D. *On Death and Dying*. New York: Macmillan, 1969.

Lacher, Mortimer J., M.D., and John R. Redman, M.D. *Hodgkin's Disease: The Consequences of Survival*. Philadelphia: Lea & Febiger, 1990.

Lansky, Shirley B., M.D., Marcy A. List, Ph.D., and Chris Ritter-Sterr, M.S. "Psychosocial Consequences of Cure." *Cancer* 58 (1986): 529–533.

Laufer, Robert S., M. S. Gallops, and Ellen Frey-Wouters. "War Stress and Trauma: The Vietnam Veteran Experience." *Journal of Health and Social Behavior* 25 (March 1984): 65–85.

Leerhsen, Charles, with Shawn D. Lewis et al. "Unite and Conquer." *Newsweek*, February 5, 1990.

Leporrier, Michel, M.D., et al. "A New Technique to Protect Ovarian Function Before Pelvic Irradiation." *Cancer* 60 (1987): 2201–2204.

Lerner, Harriet Goldhor, Ph.D. *The Dance of Anger: A Woman's Guide to Changing the Patterns of Intimate Relationships.* New York: Harper & Row, 1986.

Levitt, Paul M., and Elissa S. Guralnick. *You Can Make It Back.* New York: Facts on File Publications, 1985.

Lifton, Robert Jay. *Home from the War.* New York: Simon & Schuster, 1973.

Lipson, Benjamin. *How to Collect More on Your Insurance Claims.* New York: Simon & Schuster, 1985.

Ludtke, Melissa. "Can the Mind Help Cure Disease?" *Time*, March 12, 1990.

Mathiessen, Constance. "Unsurance." *Hippocrates*, November/December 1989.

McKhann, Charles F., M.D. *The Facts About Cancer.* New York: Prentice-Hall, 1981.

Meadows, Anna T., M.D., and Wendy L. Hobbie. "The Medical Consequences of Cure." *Cancer* 58 (1986): 524–528.

Menning, Barbara Eck. "The Infertile Couple: A Plea for Advocacy." *Child Welfare* 54 (June 1975): 454-460.

Monmaney, Terrence, and Eduardo Levy-Spira with Mary Hager. "Young Survivors in a Deadly War." *Newsweek*, July 18, 1988.

Morra, Marion, and Eve Potts. *Triumph: Getting Back to Normal When You Have Cancer.* New York: Avon, 1990.

Mullan, Fitzhugh, M.D. "The Cancer Consort: Making Cancer Survivors a Positive Political Force." *Journal of Psychosocial Oncology* 5 (Spring 1987): 81–87.

———. "Needed: An Agenda for Survivors." *Cope*, November 1986.

———. "Seasons of Survival: Reflections of a Physician with Cancer." *New England Journal of Medicine* 313 (1985): 270–273.

Nader, Ralph, and Wesley J. Smith. *Winning the Insurance Game.* New York: Knightsbridge, 1990.

Northouse, Laurel L. "Living with Cancer." *American Journal of Nursing* (May 1981): 961–962.

Parachini, Allan. "Cancer Survivors: Coping with Life." *Los Angeles Times*, September 1, 1985, sec. 6.

Patterson, James T. *The Dread Disease: Cancer and Modern American Culture.* Cambridge: Harvard University Press, 1987.

Redman, John R., et al. "Semen Cryopreservation and Artificial Insemination for Hodgkin's Disease." *Journal of Clinical Oncology* 5 (February 1987): 233–238.

Podrasky, Patricia Anne. "The Family Perspective of the Cured Patient." *Cancer* 58 (1986): 522–523.

Rieker, Patricia P., Susan D. Edbril, and Marc B. Garnick. "Curative Testis Cancer Therapy: Psychosocial Sequelae." *Journal of Clinical Oncology* 3 (August 1985): 1117–1126.

Roberts, Leslie. *Cancer Today: Origins, Prevention, and Treatment.* Washington, D.C.: National Academy Press, 1984.

Roemer, Ruth, M.D. "The Right to Health Care — Gains and Gaps." *American Journal of Public Health* 78 (March 1988): 241–247.

Rosenbaum, Ernest H., M.D., and Isadora R. Rosenbaum. *A Comprehensive Guide for Cancer Patients and Their Families.* Palo Alto: Bull Publishing, 1980.

Rosenthal, Elisabeth. "The Cancer War: A Major Advance." *New York Times Magazine,* October 8, 1989.

Sattilaro, Anthony J., M.D., and Thomas J. Monte. *Recalled by Life.* Boston: Houghton Mifflin, 1982.

Scarf, Maggie. *Intimate Partners: Patterns in Love and Marriage.* New York: Random House, 1987.

Segal, Julius, Ph.D. *Winning Life's Toughest Battles.* New York: Ivy Books, 1986.

Shapiro, Joseph P. "Liberation Day for the Disabled." *U.S. News & World Report,* September 18, 1989.

Siegel, Mary-Ellen. *The Cancer Patient's Handbook.* New York: Walker, 1986.

Silberner, Joanne. "First, You Beat the Cancer." *U.S. News & World Report,* November 6, 1989.

Simonton, Stephanie Matthews. *The Healing Family.* New York: Bantam, 1984.

Slaby, Andrew E., M.D. *Aftershock.* New York: Villard, 1989.

Smedes, Lewis B. *Forgive and Forget: Healing the Hurts We Don't Deserve.* San Francisco: Harper & Row, 1984.

Sontag, Susan. *Illness as Metaphor.* New York: Farrar, Straus & Giroux, 1977.

Sourkes, Barbara M., Ph.D. *The Deepening Shade.* Pittsburgh: University of Pittsburgh Press, 1982.

Tucker, M. A., M.D., et al. "Risk of Second Cancers After Treatment for Hodgkin's Disease." *New England Journal of Medicine* 318 (1988): 76–81.

U.S. Department of Education. Office of Special Education and Rehabilitative Services. *Summary of Existing Legislation Affecting Per-*

sons with Disabilities. Publication no. E-88-22014, 1988.
U.S. Department of Health and Human Services. National Institutes of Health. *After Breast Cancer: A Guide to Followup Care.* NIH publication no. 87-2400, 1987.
Veninga, Robert. *A Gift of Hope: How We Survive Our Tragedies.* Boston: Little, Brown, 1985.
Viorst, Judith. *Necessary Losses.* New York: Ballantine, 1986.

If you would like to start a local chapter of Cancervive, please contact:

CANCERVIVE, INC.
6500 Wilshire Boulevard, Suite 500
Los Angeles, California 90048
(213) 203-9232